AF796687

With compliments

SCHWARZ
PHARMA

M. Safar · M. Stimpel · A. Zanchetti (Eds.)

Hypertension in Postmenopausal Women

With 21 Figures

Springer-Verlag
Berlin Heidelberg New York
London Paris Tokyo
Hong Kong Barcelona
Budapest

Michel Emile Safar, M.D.
Professor of Therapeutics, Department of Internal Medicine 1, and Hypertension Research Center, Hôpital Broussais, F–75674 Paris Cedex 14, France

Michael Stimpel, M.D.
Assistant Professor of Medicine, Medical School, University of Cologne, D-50931 Cologne, and Schwarz Pharma AG, Department of Clinical Research, D–40789 Monheim, Germany

Alberto Zanchetti, M.D.
Professor of Medicine, Centro di Fisiologia, Clinica e Ipertensione, Policlinico, I–20122 Milano, Italy

ISBN 3-540-58144-8 Springer-Verlag Berlin Heidelberg New York
ISBN 0-387-58144-8 Springer-Verlag Berlin Heidelberg New York

Typesetting: Mitterweger Plankstadt
21/3130-5 4 3 2 1 – Printed on acid-free paper

Contents

List of Contributors

ANTOON AMERY, M.D., Ph.D., FRCP (Edin)
Hypertension and Cardiovascular Rehabilitation Unit, Department of Molecular and Cardiovascular Research, University of Leuven, Herestraat 49, B–3000 Leuven, Belgium

VERA BITTNER, M.D.,
Division of Cardiovascular Disease, Department of Medicine, The University of Alabama at Birmingham, Birmingham, AL 35294, USA

KAREN BRADSHAW, M.D.
Assistant Professor of Obstetrics, Gynecology, and Surgery, The University of Texas, Southwestern Medical Center, Division of Reproductive Endocrinology, 5323 Harry Hines Boulevard, Dallas, TX 75235-8899, USA

HANS R. BRUNNER, M.D.
Professor of Medicine, Hypertension Division, Centre Hospitalier, Universitaire Vaudois (CHUV), CH–1101 Lausanne, Switzerland

CRISTOPHER J. BULPITT, M.D., MSc.
Division of Geriatric Medicine, Department of Medicine, Royal Postgraduate Medical School, Hammersmith Hospital, London W12 ONN, United Kingdom

JEAN M. CACCIABAUDO, M.D.
Clinical Fellow in Hypertension and Cardiology, The New York Hospital Cornell Medical Center, Starr 4, 525 East 68th Street, New York, NY 10021, USA

ROBERT FAGARD, M.D., PH.D.
Hypertension and Cardiovascular Rehabilitation Unit, Department of Molecular and Cardiovascular Research, University of Leuven, Herestraat 49, B–3000 Leuven, Belgium

PAUL LIJNEN, M.D., PH.D.
Hypertension and Cardiovascular Rehabilitation Unit, Department of Molecular and Cardiovascular Research, University of Leuven, Herestraat 49, B–3000 Leuven, Belgium

ROGERIO A. LOBO, M.D.
Professor of Obstetrics and Gynecology, University of Southern California, Room 1M2, Women's Hospital, LAC & USC Medical Center, Los Angeles, CA 90033, USA

KARIN MANHEM, M.D., PH.D.
Department of Medicine CK2, Östra Hospital, S–416 85 Göteborg, Sweden

SUZANNE OPARIL, M.D.
Professor of Medicine, The University of Alabama at Birmingham, 1034 Zeigler Research Building, 703 South 19th Street, UAB Station, Birmingham, AL 35294–0007, USA

JEAN E. SEALEY, M.D.
Professor of Medicine, Cardiovascular Center, The New York Hospital, Cornell Medical Center, Starr 4, 525 East 68th Street, New York, NY 10021, USA

JAN A. STAESSEN, M.D., PH.D.
Hypertension and Cardiovascular Rehabilitation Unit, Department of Molecular and Cardiovascular Research, University of Leuven, Herestraat 49, B–3000 Leuven, Belgium

ALBERTO ZANCHETTI, M.D.
Professor of Medicine, Centro die Fisiologia, Clinica e Ipertensione, Policlinico Via F. Sforza 35, I–20122 Milano, Italy

ANNE ZANCHI, M.D.
Hypertension Division, Centre Hospitalier, Universitaire Vaudois (CHUV), CH–1101 Lausanne, Switzerland

Introduction

ALBERTO ZANCHETTI

The meeting on hypertension in postmenopausal women, held in Monte Carlo in the context of the Third International Forum for the Evaluation of Cardiovascular Care (IFECC III), was particularly timely, as it has been among the first and few ones addressing the attention of both clinical investigators and practicing doctors to a field largely disregarded for many years. Apart from recognizing that blood pressure is frequently increasing in women around the menopausal age and that the overall cardiovascular risk rises after the menopause, until recently no concerted action was devoted to better clarify the multiple relations between hormonal status, blood pressure, risk, cardiovascular complications and prevention in a condition in which women spend one third of their lives.

The meeting in Monte Carlo, the proceedings of which are here published, testifies to a new attention to these problems. Increased knowledge is not synonimous of increased understanding, however. In fact, if we now know that the higher incidence of hypertension after the menopause is not a mere effect of passing age, but is the result of a greater steepness of the age-related blood pressure increase around the menopausal period, we are still ignorant of the mechanisms underlying this phenomenon. The mechanisms of the increased cardiovascular risk of postmenopausal women are also uncertain, and even the mounting evidence of a cardiovascular protective effect of hormonal replacement therapy, though clinically attractive, has added new problems to old ones. As the use of hormonal replacement therapy becomes more and more widespread, we would like to know more about the mechanisms of this protection, and to better appreciate its limits, if any limits occur. The multiple interference of hormonal replacement therapy with cardiovascular control mechanisms should be explored in greater depth, in particular with the renin-angiotensin system and with endothelium function, both of which play such an important role in hypertension.

At a time when due emphasis is placed on the need of individualized antihypertensive therapy, with specific recommendations for the hypertensive patient with diabetes, that with dyslipidemia, that with one or another target organ involvement, it may also be necessary to think of specific recommendations for this large subset of the hypertensive population, the postmenopausal hypertensive women and perhaps, separately, the postmenopausal hypertensive women with hormonal replacement therapy.

If we do not have the answer now, this does not detract from the importance of the problem that requires more research and other meetings such as the one reported here. I am particularly grateful to all the contributors that made the Monte Carlo meeting so stimulating and make this volume of such a great interest to a large medical audience. I am also grateful to Schwarz Pharma that generously supported the meeting in Monte Carlo and the publication of this volume.

Cardiovascular Risk in Postmenopausal Women: What is Known and what is Unknown

Karin Manhem

Introduction

The leading causes of death in postmenopausal women in the United States are coronary heart disease (CHD) and stroke, despite a steady decline during the past two decades [1, 2]. Cardiovascular disease (CVD) secondary to atherosclerosis occurs in much lower frequencies in many third world countries, as well as in several oriental populations [3]. The prevalence of CVD in premenopausal women is reflected by between a fifth and half as many deaths in CHD below the age of 50–55 years, as in men of the same age. After menopause, women develop CHD at the same rate as men, although approximately 6–10 years later [4]. The incidence of stroke is increased with age in both sexes, and most types of stroke are slightly more common in men than in women [5]. Despite the impact of CVD on postmenopausal womens' health, very few population-based studies of CVD have included women, or focused exclusively on women. Furthermore, few clinical trials have involved female populations large enough to allow adequate evaluation of treatments for CVD in women [2].

It is generally believed that women lose their cardiovascular advantage after menopause, and Framingham data suggests that there might be an effect of menopause [6]. However, statistical data does not offer strong support for the hypothesis that menopause per se is accompanied by a rise in the risk of coronary disease [1, 7]. A moderate effect of menopause could easily be lost in population statistics, since individual age at natural menopause varies with about a decade [1]. In contrast to natural menopause, bilateral oophorectomy produces an evident risk for coronary disease [6, 8, 9]. There are also important coronary risk factors that affect onset of menopause. Smoking contributes quite strongly to early menopause, while obesity, on the other hand tends to result in delayed menopause [1]. Most studies show an increased risk of heart disease in women with early menopause, but the results are at variance [10]. Studies of CVD risk by parity show mixed results and are difficult to interpret since social class does influence both CVD and number of pregnancies [10]. The influence of age at menarche on the risk of CVD is not well documented [10].

Estrogen and Cardiovascular Risk in Postmenopausal Women

The observation that premenopausal women to some degree are "protected" from CVD raises the question of a positive effect of estrogen on the cardiovascular system. Population studies suggest an association between androgenic activity and increased risk of CHD [11]. Exogenous estrogens given as replacement therapy differ in type, dose and composition from estrogen in oral contraceptives (OC) [2]. Three large prospective studies have examined the influence of postmenopausal estrogen use on CVD: the Framingham study of 1234 women aged 53–83 years, the Nurses' Health Study (NHS) of 32 317 women aged 30–50 years, and the Lipid Research Clinic Study (LRCS) of 2269 women aged 40–69. Unopposed oral estrogen given postmenopausally has been shown to reduce the risk of coronary events by about 50 % [12]. In a recent report, estrogen replacement therapy was associated with an 87 % reduction of coronary artery disease in postmenopausel women undergoing coronary angiography [13]. The benefit of estrogen is most pronounced among current and recent users, and while the beneficial effects do not seem to vary with duration of treatment, variations with dose and age of the patient are possible [14]. Estrogen use has not previously been proven to affect the risk of stroke [8], but in a recent report from Sweden, hormone replacement therapy with estrogen, alone or in combination with cyclical progestins, reduced the risk of stroke substantially [15]. The effect of addition of progestins to estrogen is less well studied. In a population-based investigation including almost 5000 participants, Nabulsi et al. found a protective effect on CVD after progestin addition [16]. Noteworthy is that the women receiving estrogen are healthier, more aware of their health, and visit their doctors more often than other women [12], but substantial data suggests that no more than a fraction of the benefit of estrogen can be explained by this [14].

Oral contraceptives are associated with an increased risk of heart disease and venous as well as arterial thromboembolic episodes, especially in older premenopausal women and particularly those who smoke [10, 17]. This is true for present but not for previous users [10]. Postmortem examinations show that CVD usually is thromboembolic rather than atheroembolic [18]. The estrogen to progestin ratio is of importance since estrogen and progestin have opposed effects on the lipid levels [19].

Traditional Cardiovascular Risk Factors

Age

Age is a powerful predictor of CVD in women and men, but the onset of disorder occurs approximately 10 years later in women [20]. After 50 years of age, a sevenfold increase in CVD mortality in women was observed for each 10-year age increment in the LRCS follow-up study [21]. However, at any age men show a higher incidence of CVD than women [2]. A nonsignificant trend towards a decreasing benefit of estrogen on coronary disease with increasing age was found in the 10-year follow-up from the NHS, consistent with Framingham data [8]. It is speculated on the other hand, that estrogen has an increasing protective effect on the risk of stroke with advancing age [22]. Moreover, age is accompanied with several resetting in the cardiovascular system, such as decreased baroreceptor sensitivity and reduction of receptor reactivity to β-adrenergic neurotransmitters. Furthermere, heart rate reactivity to sympathetic stimuli is impaired, and vagal tonus is increased with age [23].

Hypertension

Hypertension is one of the main risk factors for CVD in women and men [20]. In elderly women it is the single most important factor [24]. The prevalence is higher in men than in women before the age ot 35 years, but by the age of 65 the prevalence is higher in women [25]. Morbidity and mortality rates at any blood pressure level are higher in men, and hypertensive women appear to have better prognosis than men [216]. The benefit of antihypertensive treatment may not be as large in women as in men [27], but this conclusion might be a result of inadequate samples [28]. The effect of menopause on blood pressure is difficult to evaluate since menopause as well as blood pressure are influenced by factors such as body mass index (BMI), socioeconomic class, and smoking [29]. However, Staessen et al. found that menopause may be accompanied by a steeper rise in SBP [29]. This was also found by Bonithon-Kopp et al. in a cross-sectional study of 435 women aged 45–54 [7]. Posner et al. did find higher SBP in postmenopausal compared to premenopausal women in a recent report from the Framingham study [30]. No effect of menopause on blood pressure was found at the initial Framingham examination [31]. In a recent review by Barrett-Connor and Bush, it is stated that replacement therapy is associated with a lower blood pressure [10]. According to the Framingham study, the NHS, and the LRCS, the prevalence of hypertension was not influenced by estrogen use [27]. OC raise the blood pressure in most women, but development of true hypertension is uncommon [27]. In essential hypertension, changes in sex steroids are shown in both men and women [32]. The hemodynamic pattern differs between hypertensive men and premenopausal women, with increased resting heart rate, cardiac index and pulse pressure combined with lower total peripheral resistance in the women than in the men [33].

Glucose Intolerance / Hyperinsulinemia and Diabetes Mellitus

Regarding diabetes, prospective and case-control studies have shown an increased risk of CVD both in women and men, but the risk is considerably higher among diabetic women [4, 20]. The incidence of CVD in diabetic women is almost three times that of nondiabetic women, while the diabetic men have roughly twice the risk of nondiabetic men [28]. Furthermore, in the Framingham study, glucose intolerance was found to be an independent risk factor for cardiovascular mortality in women [4]. Diabetic women had the same risk of myocardial infarction as nondiabetic men of the same age [4]. This could partly be explained by an increase of other risk factors among these women, such as hypertension, obesity and increased cholesterol and triglyceride values [20]. An increase in insulin associated with menopause was reported by Razay and coworkers, and is in concordance with Framingham data, where higher rates of glucose intolerance were found in postmenopausal women [30, 34]. However, other studies have failed to show any change in blood glucose in women after menopause [7, 31]. Cross-sectional studies suggest a lowering effect on both insulin and glucose due to estrogen use [35], whereas OC causes impaired glucose tolerance [36]. Progestin-only OC have no effect on carbohydrate metabolism [36].

Blood Lipids

Total cholesterol and HDL cholesterol both have a major impact on womens' risk of CVD, but opinions differ regarding the role of LDL cholesterol [2]. In the Lipid Research Clinics follow-up study, total chlesterol did not predict CHD mortality in women, neither did LDL cholesterol, but triglyceride levels and HDL appeared to be strong predictors [21]. In the Framingham study, total cholesterol and LDL were independent risk factors in women and men, elevated triglycerides was an independent risk in women only, and HDL had a substantial impact on CHD irrespective of level of total plasma cholesterol [37]. Thus, age and sex are important determinants of lipids and lipoproteins [38]. After menopause, a change in lipids with increased cholesterol levels occurs within 2 years of menopause [7]. There are studies suggesting that women in Western Societies and Japan experience this change at menopause in contrast to women in Third World countries [7]. By the age of 50, higher total cholesterol and LDL levels are found, triglycerides and VLDL concentrations approach those in men, but HDL remains by contrast significantly higher in women throughout life [38]. The increments in lipid status have been found following both natural and surgical menopause as compared to age-matched controls [38]. Recent data from the Framingham offspring study show 8 % higher values (although not statistically significant) of Lipoprotein(a) in postmenopausal compared to premenopausal women [39]. The effect of menopause on lipid levels is strong in contrast to other CV risk factors such as hypertension, body weight, smoking habits, and glucose intolerance [38]. Although it is plausible that lipid modification is protective also in women, most intervention studies have been performed in men, and the preventive effect of lipid modification in women may be different [38]. Other studies are less consistent regarding an increased risk of disease among with cholesterol concentrations of 200–240 mg/dl [2]. It is believed that approximately 50 % of the positive effect of estrogen replacement hormone therapy is caused by alterations in lipids, increased HDL, decreased LDL, and decreased total cholesterol [10, 38]. In a recent randomized trial, Nabulsi and coworkers found higher levels of HDL subfractions (lipoprotein 2 and 3 and apolipoptotein A-I) in users compared to nonusers [16]. It is suggested that percutaneous administration have a weaker effect on VLDL and LDL levels [40]. Addition of progesteron to postmenopausal estrogen may induce changes in serum lipid and lipoproteins which are opposite to those observed with estrogen, and the triglyceride reducing capacity seems favorable [38, 40]. The fact that combined OC cause increase in LDL, and in particular in triglycerides seem to be related to the androgenicity of the progestin, the net effect on HDL depends on the balance estrogen/progestins [36].

Obesity

Whether obesity alone is an independent risk factor for CHD remains unclear, but Framingham data suggests this, and emphasizes that this is particularly pronounced in younger women [41]. The distribution of body fat with increased waist to hip (W/H) ratio was an independent risk factor for AMI, angina, stroke, and overall mortality in women in the 12-year follow up of participants in the study of women in Göteborg [42]. Obesity is often accompanied by other risk factors, i.e. diabetes, increased lipid levels, and hypertension [43]. Sex hormone-binding globulin (SHBG), a major determinant of the ratio of free to bound plasma to testosterone, has been found to be significantly associated with the BMI and W/H ratio, indicating that an unfavorable fat distribution is associated with increased androgenicity [44]. The conversion of androstendione to estrone occurs in adipose tissue [10]. One might speculate whether leaner women have lower levels of endogenous estrogen and thereby experience an increased risk of CVD, since thinner women tend to benefit more from replacement therapy [8].

Smoking

Smoking is an important risk factor in women and men [2]. In younger women smoking is a major risk factor for AMI, but the contribution of smoking to the risk of CVD is greater in men [20]. Smokers experience an earlier menopause [1], and smoking is believed to exert an antiestrogenic effect on the cardiovascular system [45]. Furthermore, smoking is also associated with decreased HDL levels, increased platelet aggregability, and elevated fibrinogen levels [20]. Smokers are leaner, and this may as previously noted be associated with lower estrogen levels. The impact of this on CVD is not known.

Fibrinogen, Clotting Factors, and Platelet Activity

Fibrinogen is a powerful predictor of CHD in women and men [46]. In men, factor VII coagulant activity and factor VII antigen are associated with risk of ischemic heart disease [46]. Scarabin and coworkers found an increased level of both factor VIIc and factor VIIag in postmenopausal compared to premenopausal women [47]. The effect of menopause on fibrinogen is not well documented, and when investigated, the results are at variance [7]. Platelet activity does increase with age [24], but clotting function is not essentially changed as a function of age although older women run a higher risk of thromboembolic morbidity [24]. the impact of replacement therapy on clotting and fibrinolytic system is not well documented, but unfavorable changes in fibrinogen, clotting factors and platelets after OC treatment have been documented [24, 48].

Possible Cardiovascular Risk Factors

The changes in steroid hormone levels after menopause may also influence the cardiovascular system in other ways and hence alter the risk of CVD. There might exist an interaction between sex, environmental stress and atherogenesis. This has been found in animal studies [49, 50]. Psychosocial risk factors in women are not extensively studied. From the Framingham study an association between type A behavior and CHD incidence in women has been reported [51]. An inverse relationship between education and CHD risk has also been found in women [52]. In female monkeys estrogen appears to be protective since atherosclerosis was two to ten times as extensive in ovariectomized monkeys as in menstruating animals [53, 54]. The antiatherogenetic effects of hormone replacement treatment with estrogen and the combination of estrogen and progesterone have recently been shown in this animal model [55]. An influence on central adrenergic activity by female sex hormones has been obtained both in human and in animal models [56, 57]. Another possible mechanism by which estrogen and progesterone may affect the cardiovascular system is by alteration in the peripheral alpha- or beta-adrenoreceptor sensitivity [58, 59]. Recent investigations suggest that female sex hormones may regulate contractile responses of cascular smooth muscle by modifying endothelial functions [60].

Another possible mechanism behind an estrogen effect on CHD may include direct action on the myocardium and the vessel walls where specific steroid receptors have been found [61, 62]. The effect on the endothelial cells by estrogen receptors may play a role in the local circulation and by this mechanism influence the development of the atherosclerotic plaque [63].

Activation of the renin-angiotensin system by OC is well documented [64, 65]. Estrogen stimulates the hepatic synthesis of plasma renin substrate [65]. On the contrary replacement therapy with natural estrogen alone or in combination with norethisterone acetate have been given without any effects on renin, angiotensin II or aldosterone levels [66]. Hence, steroid hormones exert specific effects on the renin-angiotensin system, but it is not well documented to what extent endogenous physiologic levels of sex hormones may influence this system.

The production of growth factors in breast cancer is affected by estrogen, and this might also be important for the cardiovascular system [67].

Summary and Conclusion

Women experience an increased risk of CVD after menopause. Early menopause and surgically induced menopause with oophorectomy does increase the risk. Diabetes even in younger postmenopausal ages and low HDL cholesterol markedly reduce the female advantage over men. Further, hypertriglyceridemia is an independent risk factor in women. The most prominent change in risk factors correlated to menopause is an impaired lipid composition. Replacement therapy reduces the risk of CVD by 25 %–50 %, mainly through improvement of the lipid composition. Other mechanisms that may decrease the risk of CVD are improved carbohydrate metabolism, a blood pressure reducing capacity and positive changes in the clotting system. Estrogen influences the sympaticoadrenal system, the renin-angiotensin system and exerts direct effects on the myocardium and large vessels. Unknown risk factors of CVD in postmenopausal women may include changes in these systems due to decreased endogenous estrogen levels.

References

1. Stampfer MJ, Colditz GA, Willet WC (1990) Menopause and heart disease. A review. Ann N Y Acad Sci 592:193–203
2. Bush T (1990) The epidemiology of cardiovascular disease in postmenopausal women. Ann N Y Acad Sci 592:263–271
3. Reeve J (1992) Future prospects for hormone replacement therapy. Br Med Bull 48:458–468
4. Castelli WP (1988) Cardiovascular disease in women. Am J Obstet Gynecol 158:1553–1560
5. Dyken ML, Wolf PA, Barnett HJM et al. (1984) Risk factors in stroke: a statement for physicians by the subcommittee on risk factors and stroke of the Stroke Council. Stroke 15:1105–1111
6. Gordon T, Kannel WB, Hjortland MC et al. (1978) Menopause and coronary heart disease: the Framingham study. Ann Intern Med 89:157–161
7. Bonithon-Kopp C, Scarabin P-Y, Darne B et al. (1990) Menopause-related changes in lipoproteins and some other cardiovascular risk factors. Int J Epidemiol 19:42–48
8. Stampfer MJ, Colditz GA, Willett WC et al. (1991) Postmenopausal estrogen therapy and cardiovascular disease. Ten-year follow-up from the nurses' health study. N Engl J Med 325:756–762
9. Parrish HM, Carr LA, Hall DG et al. (1967) Time interval from castration in premonopausal women to development of excessive coronary atherosclerosis. Am J Obstet Gynecol 99:155–162
10. Barrett-Connor E, Bush T (1991) Estrogen and coronary heart disease in women. JAMA 265:1861–1867
11. Godsland IF, Wynn V, Crook D et al. (1987) Sex, gonadal steroids and plasma lipoproteins: prevailing assumptions and unanswered questions. Am Heart J 114:1467
12. Berrett-Connor E (1992) Risks and benefits of replacement estrogen. Annu Rev Med 43:239–251
13. Hong MK, Romm PA, Reagan K et al. (1992) Effects of estrogen replacement therapy on serum lipid values and angiographically defined coronary artery disease in postmenopausal women. Am J Cardiol 69:176–178
14. Stampfer MJ, Colditz GA (1991) Estrogen replacement therapy and coronary heart disease: A quantitative assessment of the epidemiologic evidence. Prev Med 20:47–63
15. Falkeborn M, Persson I, Terent A et al. (1993) Hormone replacement therapy and risk of stroke. Arch Intern Med 153:1201–1209
16. Nabulsi AA, Folsom AR, White A et al (1993) Association of hormone-replacement therapy with various cardivascular risk factors in postmenopausal women. N Engl J Med 328:1067–1075
17. Meade TW (1988) Risks and mechanisms of cardiovascular events in users of oral contraceptives. Am J Obstet Gynecol 158:1646–1652
18. Stadel BV (1981) Oral contraceptives and cardiovascular disease. N Engl J Med 305:612–618, 672–677
19. Knopp RH (1988) Cardiovascular effects of endogenous and exogenous sex hormones over a woman's lifetime. Am J Obstet Gynecol 158:1630–1643
20. Corrao JM, Becker RC, Ockene IS et al. (1990) Coronary heart disease risk factors in women. Cardiology 77[Suppl 2]:8–24
21. Bush TL, Criqui MN, Cowan LD et al. (1987) Cardiovascular disease mortality in women: results from the Lipid Research Clinics Follow-up Study. In: Eaker ED, Packard B, Wenger NK et al. (eds) Coronary heart disease in women. Proceedings of an NIH workshop. Haymarket Doyma, New York, pp 106–111

22. Paganini-Hill A, Ross RK, Henderson BE (1988) Postmenopausal oestrogen treatment and stroke: a prospective study. BMJ 297:519–522
23. Weisfelt ML (1985) The aging heart. Hosp Pract 20:115–119
24. Tepper R, Goldberger S, May JY et al. (1992) Hormonal replacement therapy in postmenopausal women and cardiovascular disease: an overview. Obstet Gynecol Surv 47:426–431
25. Rowland M, Roberts J (1982) Blood pressure levels of persons 6–74 years: United States 1976–1980. National health and Nutrition Examination Survey II. NCHS advance data. Vital and Health Statistics of the National Center for Health Statistics. no 84. US Department of Health and Human Services Washington
26. Lerner DJ, Kannel WB (1986) Patterns of coronary heart disease morbidity and mortality in the sexes: a 26-year follow-up of the Framingham population. Am Heart J 111:383–390
27. Hall PM (1990) Hypertension in women. Cardiology 77[Suppl 2]:25–30
28. Kannel WB, Doyle JT, Ostfeld AM et al. (1984) Optimal resources for primary prevention of atherosclerotic diseases. Circulation 70:157A–205A
29. Staessen J, Bulpitt CJ, Fagard R et al. (1989) The influence of menopause on blood pressure. J Hum Hypertens 3:427–433
30. Posner BM, Cupples LA, Miller DR et al. (1993) Diet, menopause, and serum cholesterol levels in women: the Framingham study. Am Heart J 125:483–489
31. Hjortland MC, McNamara PM, Kannel WB (1976) Some atherogenetic concommitants of menopause: the Framingham Study. Am J Epidemiol 103:304–311
32. Hughes GS, Mathur RS, Margolius HS (1989) Sex steroid hormones are altered in essential hypertension. J Hypertens 7:181–187
33. Messerli FH, Garavaglia GE, Schmieder RE et al (1987) Disparate cardiovascular findings in men and women with essential hypertension. Ann Intern Med 107:158–161
34. Razay G, Heaton KW, Bolton CH (1992) Coronary heart disease risk factors in relation to the menopause. Q J Med 85:889–896
35. Bush TL, Miller VT (1987) Effects of pharmacologic agents used during menopause: impact on lipids and lipoproteins. In: Mishell DR (ed) Menopause: physiology and pharmacology. Year Book Medical Publishers, Chicago, pp 187–208
36. Crook D, Godsland IF, Wynn V (1988) Oral contraceptives and coronary heart disease: modulation of glucose tolerance and plasma lipid risk factors by progestins. Am J Obstet Gynecol 158:1612–1620
37. Castelli WP, Garrison RJ, Wilson PWF et al. (1986) Incidence of coronary heart disease and lipoprotein cholesterol levels: the Framingham Study. JAMA 256:2835–2838
38. Jensen J (1991) Effects of sex steroids on serum lipids and lipoproteins. Baillieres Clin Obstet Gynaecol 5:867–887
39. Jenner JL, Ordovas JM, Lamon-Fava S et al. (1993) Effects of age, sex, and menopausal status on plasma lipoprotein(a) levels. Circulation 87:1135–1141
40. Moorjani S, Dupont A, Labrie F et al. (1991) Changes in plasma lipoprotein and apolipoprotein composition in relation to oral versus percutaneus administration of estrogen alone or in cyclic association with Ultrogestan in menopausal women. J Clin Endocrinol Metabol 73:373–377
41. Hubert HB, Feinleib M, McNamara PM et al. (1983) Obesity as an independent risk factor for cardiovascular disease: a 26-year follow-up of participants in the Framingham Study. Circulation 67:968–976
42. Lapidus L, Bengtsson C, Larsson B et al. (1984) Distribution of adipose tissue and risk of CVD and death: a 12-year follow-up of participants in the study of women in Göteborg, Sweden. BMJ 289:1257–1261
43. Kafrissen ME (1990) Prevention of cardiovascular risk in women. A new concern for the obstetrician/gynecologist. Acta Obstet Gynecol Scand Suppl 152:13–20

44. Haffner SM, Katz MS, Dunn JF (1991) Increased upper body and overall adiposity is associated with decreased sex hormone binding globulin in postmenopausal women. Int J Obes 15:471–478
45. Khaw KT, Tazuke S, Barrett-Connor E (1988) Cigarette smoking and levels of adrenal androgens in postmenopausal women. N Engl J Med 318:1705–1708
46. Meade TW, Mellows S, Brozovic M et al. (1986) Haemostatic function and ischemic heart disease: principal results of the Northwick Park Heart Study. Lancet 2:533–537
47. Scarabin PV, Bonithon-Kopp C, Bara L et al. (1990) Factor VI activation and menopausal status. Thromb Res 57:227–234
48. Meade TW, Brozović M, Chakrabarti R et al. (1976) An epidemiological study of the haemostatic and other effects of oral contraceptives. Br J Haematol 34:353–364
49. Kaplan JR, Manuck SB, Clarkson TB et al. (1982) Social status, environment, and atherosclerosis in cynomolgus monkeys. Atherosclerosis 2:359–368
50. Schneiderman N (1987) Psychophysiologic factors in atherogenesis and coronary artery disease. Circulation 76[Suppl I]:1–47
51. Haynes SG, Feinleib M, Kannel WB (1980) The relationship of psychosocial factors to CHD in the Framingham Study. Am J Epidemiol 111:37–58
52. Jacobsen BK, Thelle DS (1988) Risk factors for coronary heart disease and level of education. Am J Epidemiol 127:923–932
53. Clarkson TB, Adams MR, Kaplan JR et al. (1989) From menarche to menopause: coronary artery atherosclerosis and protection in cynomolgus monkeys. Am J Obstet Gynecol 160:1280–1285
54. Adams MR, Kaplan JR, Clarkson TB et al. (1985) Ovariectomy, social status, and atherosclerosis in cynomolgus monkeys. Atherosclerosis 5:192–200
55. Adams MR, Kaplan JR, Manuck SB et al. (1990) Inhibition of coronary atherosclerosis by 17-beta estradiol in ovariectomizes monkeys. Atherosclerosis 10:1051–1057
56. Janowsky DS, Davis JM (1970) Progesterone-estrogen effects on uptake and release of norepinephrine by synaptosomes. Life Sci 9:525–531
57. Klaiber EL, Kobayashi Y, Broverman DM et al. (1971) Plasma monoamine oxidase activity in regularly menstruating women and in amenorrheic women receiving cyclic treatment with estrogens and a progestin. J Clin Endocr 33:630–638
58. Ford SP, Reynolds LP (1983) Role of adrenergic receptors in mediating estradiol-17 β-stimulated increases in uterine blood flow of cows. J Anim Sci 57:665–672
59. Rosen SG, Berk MA, Popp DA et al. (1984) β2- and α2-adrenergic receptors and receptor coupling to adenylate cyclase in human mononuclear leukocytes and platelets in relation to physiological variations of sex steroids. J Clin Endocrinol Metab 58:1068–1076
60. Zhang A, Altura BT, Altura BM (1992) Endothelial-dependent sexual dimorphism in vascular smooth muscle: role of Mg^{2+} and Na^{+}. Br J Pharmacol 105:305–310
61. McGill HC (1989) Sex steroid hormone receptors in the cardiovascular system. Postgrad Med 64–68
62. Stumpf W, Sar M (1977) The heart: a target organ for estradiol. Science 196:319–321
63. Colburn P, Buonassisi V (1978) Estrogen-binding sites in endothelial cell culture. Science 201:817–819
64. Magness RR, Rosenfeld CR (1989) Local and systemic estradiol-17 β: effects on uterine and systemic vasodilation. Am J Physiol 257 (Endocrinol Metab 19):E526–E542
65. Woods JW (1988) Oral contraceptives and hypertension. Hypertension 11[Suppl II]:II–11–II–15

66. Jespersen CM, Arnung K, Hagen C et al. (1983) Effects of natural oestrogen therapy on blood pressure and renin-angiotensin system in normotensive and hypertensive menopausal women. J Hypertens 1:361–364
67. Lippman ME, Bates S, Huff KK et al. (1987) Estrogens regulate production of specific growth factors in hormone-dependent human breast cancer. J Lab Clin Med 109:230–235

The Influence of Menopause on Blood Pressure

Jan A. Staessen, Christopher J. Bulpitt, Robert Fagard, Paul Lijnen, and Antoon Amery

Introduction

The association between menopause and the risk of cardiovascular disease has been reported to be positive by most [1–4] though not all [5] investigators. Hypertension is one of the main cardiovascular risk factors, which might explain the excess cardiovascular morbidity and mortality in post- compared with premenopausal women. Indeed, in most countries with a Western lifestyle, such as Belgium [6], men from 20 to 40 years of age have a higher systolic and diastolic blood pressure than women of similar age. In contrast, from age 55 onwards, when most women have reached menopause, the opposite tendency is observed [6]. Nonetheless, the question whether blood pressure increases independent of age following menopause has not yet been conclusively answered [7–12]. In view of the remaining uncertainty, the present study investigated whether a positive association between blood pressure and menopause was present in a random sample of the population of two Belgian districts.

Methods

A random sample of households was identified in two Belgian districts. After excluding subjects, who had recently moved or died, 3950 people were eligible, of whom 67 % took part in the study. Women from 35 to 59 years old were included in the present analysis. This age range was chosen since it embraced the extreme ages of women reporting a regular menstrual cycle or menopause.

As described in detail in previous reports [6], each household was visited twice by trained observers. At each of the two home visits five blood pressure readings in the sitting position, a pulse rate count over 1 min and a measurement of body weight and height were taken.A self-administered questionnaire was employed to inquire about the menstrual status of the female participants. Menopause was defined as the reported difinitive cessation of periods, and surgical menopause as the cessation of periods following a gynaecological operation. The questionnaire also provided information on the current use of pills containing estrogens and/or progestogens, on possible treatments with antihypertensive drugs, on smoking habits and on alcohol intake. Twenty-four-hour urine samples were analysed for sodium, potassium and creatinine.

Repeated measurements were averaged for statistical analysis. Thus each individual was characterised by the mean of ten blood pressure readings, and of two determinations of pulse rate, body weight and height. Student's *t* test was used for comparing group means. The association between hypertension and menopause across three age bands (35–41, 42–51, 52–59 years), and across two strata of body mass index, delimited by the median of the distribution (26 kg/m^2), was investigated by the method of Cochran-Mantel-Haenszel. Significant covariates of blood pressure were identified by stepwise multiple regression, terminating when all regression coefficients were significant at the 5 % level on two-tailed tests. Coincidence of regression lines was investigated by analysis of covariance, using the backward testing procedure, recommended by Kleinbaum et al. [13].

Results

Characteristics of Pre- and Postmenopausal Women

Of the 462 women, 120 had reached natural menopause. Sixty-four subjects reported that menstruation had ceased following a surgical intervention. This intervention consisted of uni- or bilateral oophorectomy combined with hysterectomy in 47 cases, and of hysterectomy not combined with oophorectomy in one subject. The exact nature of the intervention was not known in 16 women.

Pre- compared with postmenopausal subjects had a lower systolic and diastolic blood pressure (Table 1). Figure 1 shows the average systolic and diastolic blood pressure by fourths of the age distribution in premenopausal women, and in subjects with natural and surgical menopause. The rise in systolic pressure from the lowest to the upper fourth of age tended to be steeper in subjects with natural and surgical menopause than in postmenopausal women. Diastolic pressure increased along a similar line in premenopausal subjects and in women with surgical menopause, while in women with natural menopause the association of age with diastolic pressure tended to be J-shaped.

Premenopausal subjects were leaner than postmenopausal women, and had a lower urinary excretion of sodium, potassium and creatinine (Table 1).

Fig. 1. Systolic (*top*) and diastolic (*bottom*) blood pressures in fourths of the age distribution in premenopausal women (●, n = 278), and in women with natural (■, n = 120) and surgical (▲, n = 64) menopause

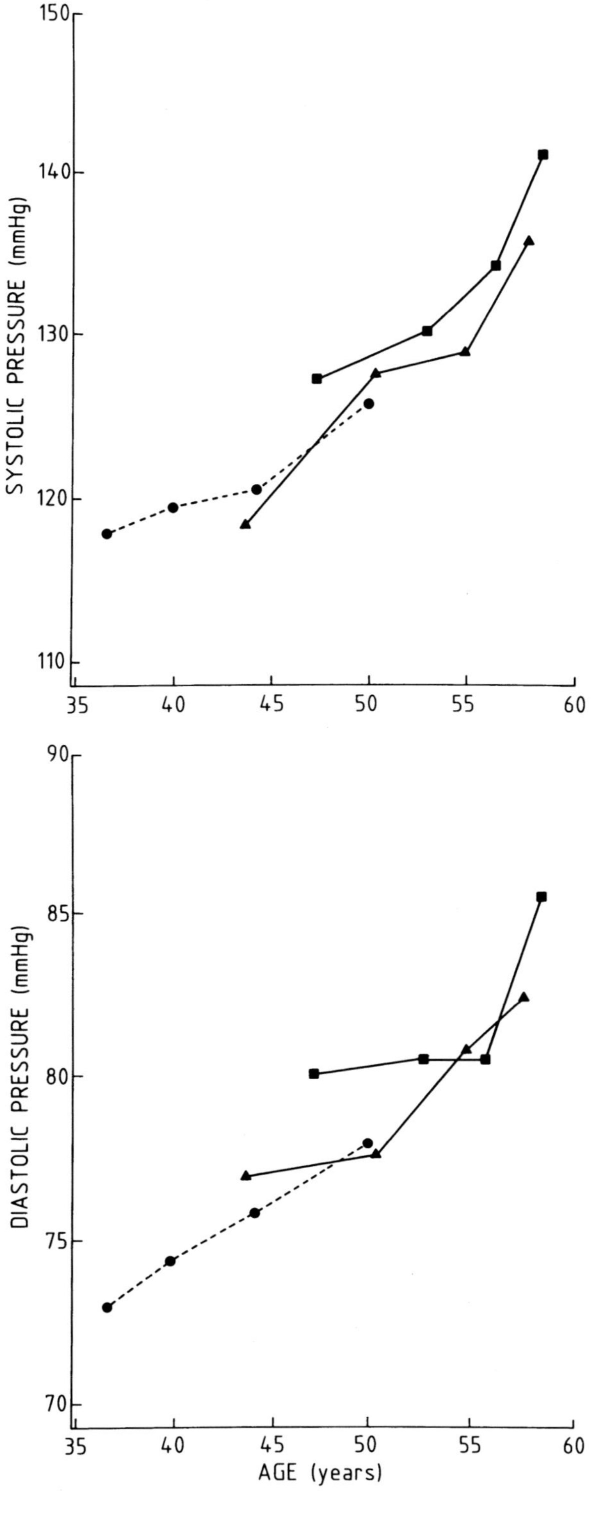
150
140
130
120
110
SYSTOLIC PRESSURE (mmHg)
35
40
45
50
55
60
90
85
80
75
70
DIASTOLIC PRESSURE (mmHg)
35
40
45
50
55
60
AGE (years)

Table 1. Characteristics of 278 pre- and 184 postmenopausal women

	Premenopausal	Postmenopausal
Age (years)	42.6 ± 5.1 (35.2–57.2)	53.0 ± 5.0*** (36.6–59.9)
Systolic pressure (mmHg)	121 ± 13 (85–194)	132 ± 17*** (97–194)
Diastolic pressure (mmHg)	75 ± 8 (52–104)	81 ± 9*** (60–121)
Pulse pressure (mmHg)	46 ± 9 (23–94)	51 ± 12*** (23–89)
Pulse rate (bpm)	75 ± 8 (51–110)	74 ± 9 (52–110)
Height (cm)	161 ± 5 (142–178)	160 ± 6 (148–176)
Body weight (kg)	66.6 ± 10.8 (44.2–105)	71.2 ± 14.1*** (47.2–131)
Body mass index (kg/m^2)	25.7 ± 4.1 (17.7–41.4)	27.9 ± 5.6*** (18.1–56.0)
Urinary volume (l/24 h)	1.48 ± 0.59 (0.22–3.80)	1.51 ± 0.58 (0.24–3.40)
Sodium (mmol/24 h)	143 ± 56 (18–360)	127 ± 59** (12–349)
Potassium (mmol/24 h)	61 ± 21 (12–171)	57 ± 17* (10–110)
Sodium:potassium ratio	2.5 ± 1.0 (0.2–8.8)	2.3 ± 1.1 (0.4–7.8)
Creatinine (mmol/24 h)	11.3 ± 2.7 (2.7–18.8)	10.3 ± 3.0*** (1.2–23.0)

Values are means ± standard deviation.
Significance of the difference between pre- and postmenopausal women: *$p < 0.05$; **$p < 0.01$; ***$p < 0.001$.

Among the 278 pre- and 184 postmenopausal women, there were 83 (43 %) and 41 (29 %) current smokers, respectively. A total of 72 subjects (23 pre- and 49 postmenopausal) were on treatment with antihypertensive medication, and 40 (39 pre- and one postmenopausal) were taking pills containing estrogens and/or progestogens.

Prevalence of Hypertension According to Menopausal Status

Hypertension, defined as having a pressure ≥ 140/90 mmHg or as being on antihypertensive treatment regardless of pressure, was more prevalent (10 % versus 40 %; $p < 0.001$) among postmenopausal women. After stratification by age and body mass index, the odds of being hypertensive for post- compared with premenopausal women were 2.2 (95 % confidence interval from 1.1 to 4.4; $p = 0.036$). When a pressure of 160/95 mmHg was used as the arbitrary cut-off point, the odds were 2.3 (1.1 to 4.6; p = 0.04).

Correlates of Blood Pressure

In stepwise multiple regression systolic and diastolic pressure were significantly and positively correlated with age, body mass index, pulse rate, taking pills with estrogens and/or progestogens and with being on antihypertensive treatment; diastolic pressure was also positively correlated with the urinary sodium:potassium ratio. Smoking, alcohol intake, and the 24-h urinary excretion of sodium and postassium were also considered for entry into the model, but were not significantly related to blood pressure.

Influence of Menopause on the Relation Between Age and Systolic Blood Pressure

Both before and after adjustment for all significant covariates, the partial correlation between systolic pressure and age was significant in premenopausal women and in women with natural and surgical menopause (Fig. 2, upper panel). Further analysis showed that the regression lines for women with natural and surgical menopause had a similar slope. However, in women with natural and surgical menopause taken together, the slope of systolic pressure on age was steeper ($p < 0.05$), and the intercept tended to be lower ($p = 0.08$) than in the premenopausal subjects (Fig. 2, upper panel).

The final regression model for all women was: systolic pressure = 60.4 – 21.5 menopause (coded 0 to 1 for condition absent and present, respectively) + 0.466 age + 0.486 interaction term between menopause and age + 0.786 body mass index + 0.266 pulse rate + 5.781 being on the pill (coded 0 or 1) + 4.794 being on antihypertensive treatment (coded 0 or 1). This model explained 29 % of the variance of systolic pressure; it indicated that the slope of systolic pressure on age was nearly 0.5 mmHg/year steeper in postmenopausal subjects. Excluding women on antihypertensive treatment and on contraceptive pills did not materially alter the regression coefficients. After these two exclusions the partial regression coefficient for age was 0.455 ($p < 0.01$) and for the interaction term between age and menopause 0.362 ($p = 0.07$).

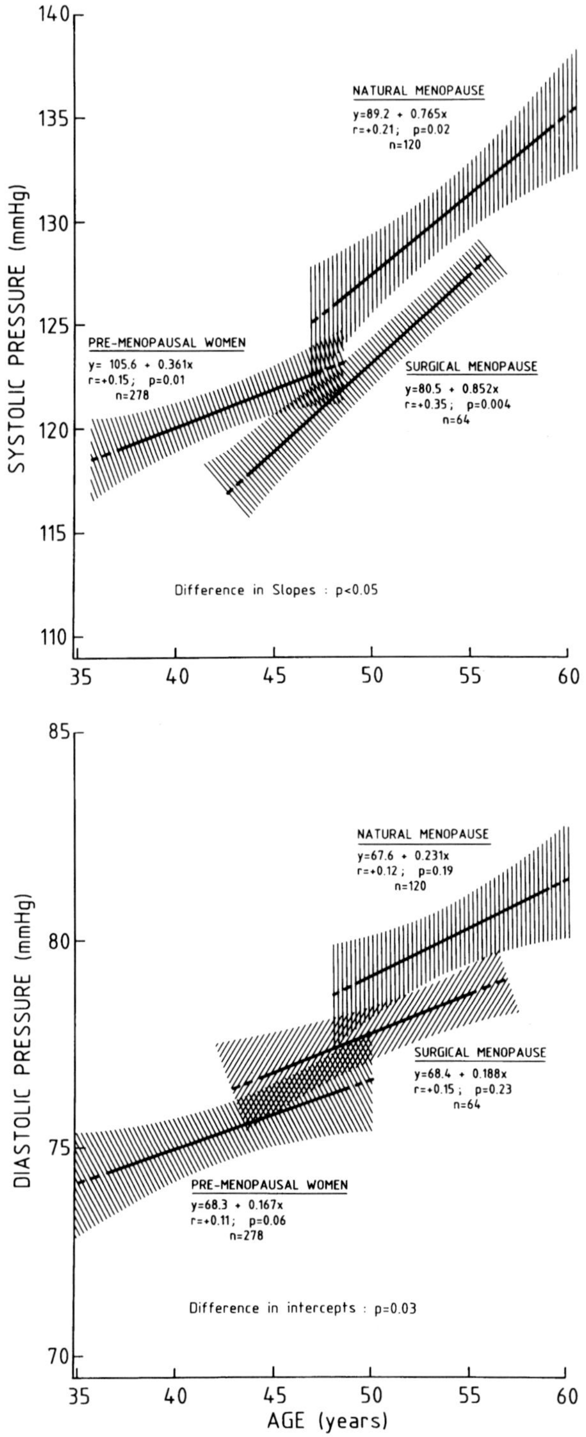

SYSTOLIC PRESSURE (mmHg)
140
135
130
125
120
115
110
NATURAL MENOPAUSE
y=89.2 + 0.765x
r=+0.21; p=0.02
n=120
PRE-MENOPAUSAL WOMEN
y= 105.6 + 0.361x
r=+0.15; p=0.01
n=278
SURGICAL MENOPAUSE
y=80.5 + 0.852x
r=+0.35; p=0.004
n=64
Difference in Slopes : p<0.05
35
40
45
50
55
60
DIASTOLIC PRESSURE (mmHg)
85
80
75
70
NATURAL MENOPAUSE
y=67.6 + 0.231x
r=+0.12; p=0.19
n=120
SURGICAL MENOPAUSE
y=68.4 + 0.188x
r=+0.15; p=0.23
n=64
PRE-MENOPAUSAL WOMEN
y=68.3 + 0.167x
r=+0.11; p=0.06
n=278
Difference in intercepts : p=0.03
AGE (years)

Influence of Menopause on the Relation Between Age and Diastolic Blood Pressure

Both before and after adjustment for all significant covariates, the partial correlation between diastolic pressure and age was significant in pre- and all postmenopausal women, but not in women with natural and surgical menopause, analysed separately (Fig. 2, lower panel). Analysis of covariance showed that there was a common and significant slope of diastolic pressure on age in women with natural and surgical menopause taken together, and in premenopausal subjects. However, the intercept of the regression line of diastolic pressure on age was on average 2.3 mmHg higher in women with natural and surgical menopause taken together, than in premenopausal subjects ($p = 0.03$). For women with natural menopause only, the upward shift in comparison with premenopausal subjects averaged 3.0 mmHg ($p < 0.03$), and for women with surgical menopause 1.2 mmHg (not significant).

The final regression model for all women was: diastolic pressure = 36.4 + 2.302 menopause (coded 0 or 1) + 0.240 age + 0.595 body mass index + 0.144 pulse rate + 0.714 urinary sodium:potassium ratio + 3.520 being on the pill (coded 0 or 1) + 1.777 being on antihypertensive treatment (coded 0 or 1). This model explained 29 % of the variance of diastolic pressure. It indicated that, independent of age and other blood pressure covariates, diastolic presure was on average 2.3 mmHg higher in post- compared with premenopausal subjects. Excluding women on antihypertensive treatment and on contraceptive pills did not materially alter the regression coefficients. After these exclusions the partial regression coefficient for age was 0.233 ($p = 0.004$) and for the effect of menopause 2.067 ($p = 0.05$).

Influence of Menopause on the Relation Between Diastolic Blood Pressure and Body Mass Index and the Sodium to Potassium Ratio

After adjustement of diastolic pressure for its significant covariates, the *t*-to-enter for the interaction term of menopause with body mass index was 2.46 ($p = 0.01$) and for the interaction with the urinary sodium: potassium ratio 2.68 ($p = 0.008$). These interactions indicated that the relationship of diastolic pressure with body mass index, or alternatively with the sodium: potassium ratio, was respectively 0.05 mmHg/kg/m^2 or 0.8 mmHg per unit steeper in post- than in premenopausal subjects (Fig. 3).

Fig. 2. Regression lines of systolic (*top*) and diastolic (*bottom*) blood pressure on age in premenopausal women and in subjects with natural or surgical menopause. The regression lines were standardised for body mass index (26.6 kg/m^2), pulse rate (74 pbm), the urinary sodium: potassium ratio (2,4), intake of the contraceptive pill (none), and antihypertensive treatment (none)

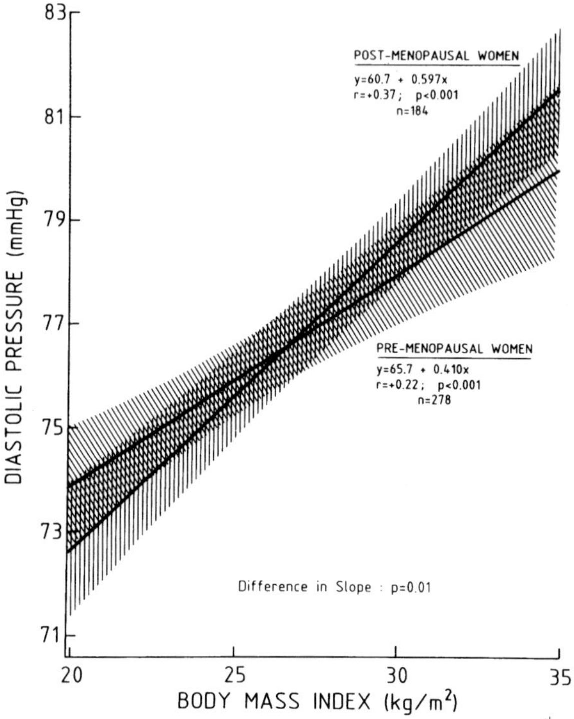
POST-MENOPAUSAL WOMEN
y=60.7 + 0.597x
r=+0.37; p<0.001
n=184
PRE-MENOPAUSAL WOMEN
y=65.7 + 0.410x
r=+0.22; p<0.001
n=278
Difference in Slope : p=0.01
DIASTOLIC PRESSURE (mmHg)
83
81
79
77
75
73
71
20
25
30
35
BODY MASS INDEX (kg/m²)

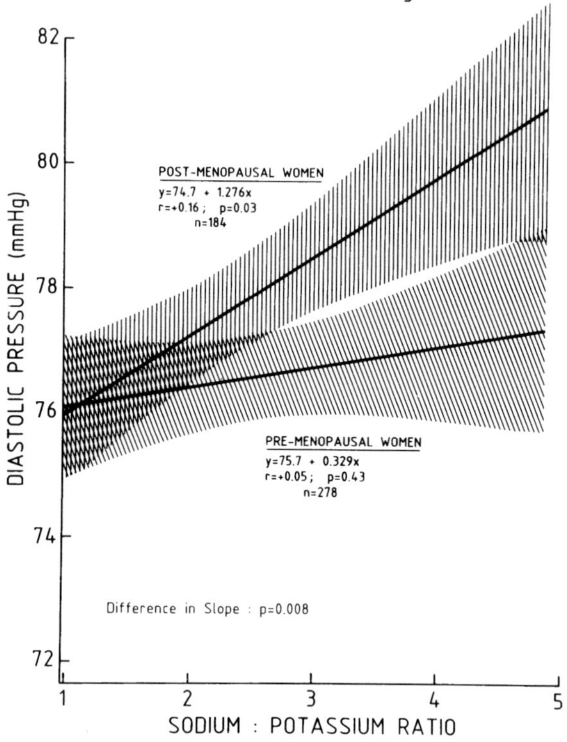
POST-MENOPAUSAL WOMEN
y=74.7 + 1.276x
r=+0.16; p=0.03
n=184
PRE-MENOPAUSAL WOMEN
y=75.7 + 0.329x
r=+0.05; p=0.43
n=278
Difference in Slope : p=0.008
DIASTOLIC PRESSURE (mmHg)
82
80
78
76
74
72
1
2
3
4
5
SODIUM : POTASSIUM RATIO

Discussion

Biological changes, occurring as a result of menopause, are difficult to evaluate, since menopause coincides with ageing, and since menopause and blood pressure are jointly influenced by factors, such as body mass index [10], socioeconomic class [12] and smoking [10]. However, multivariate statistical techniques, such as the Cochran-Mantel-Haenszel method for categorical variables, and analysis of covariance for continuous measurements, deal with the problem of confounding and have been used previously to study the effects of menopause [4]. With the use of these statistical methods the present study demonstrated that both natural and surgical menopause were associated with a 0.5 mmHg/year steeper rise in systolic pressure with age. In addition, postmenopausal women, independent of age and other covariates, had on average a 2.3 mmHg higher diastolic pressure than premenopausal subjects.

The effects of menopause on blood pressure have been assessed in previous longitudinal [8, 9] studies. Hjortland et al. [8] followed for nine biennal examinations a cohort of 1686 middle-aged women, who were premenopausal at the initial Framingham examination. They found that menopause was not accompanied by significant changes in blood pressure and body weight. However, women undergoing spontaneous menopause, were significantly leaner than their controls and this indicates that probably the menopausal subjects and their controls differed in other respects than just menstrual status alone. Weiss examined in a cross-sectional study [7] 897 women who were selected from the United States Health Examination Survey 1960–1962. This investigator found a higher diastolic pressure in postmenopausal women, while for systolic pressure a similar tendency was present in three of the four age classes. Similarly, in 539 Nigerian women, Eferakeyo and Imasuen [12] observed that menopause and postmenopausal subjects had a higher systolic and diastolic pressure than their age-matched controls, irrespective of socioeconomic class. Lindquist et al. [9–11] published a cohort study in which nearly 1000 Swedish women were followed for 6 years. Weight gain was observed in women who remained premenopausal throughout the follow-up and in women who stopped menstruating, but not in subjects who were already postmenopausal at entry into the study. Systolic and diastolic pressure rose with age and tended to increase more in the two groups for women without change in their menstrual status, than in those who had become postmenopausal [9–11].

Fig. 3. Regression lines of diastolic blood pressure on body mass index (*top*) and on the urinary sodium to potassium ratio (*bottom*) in premenopausal women and in subjects with natural or surgical menopause. The regression lines were standardised for age (47 years), body mass index (26.6 kg/m^2, *right* panel only), pulse rate (74 pbm), the urinary sodium to potassium ratio (2.4, *left* panel only), intake of the contraceptive pill (none), and antihypertensive treatment (none).

In the present study a self-administered questionnaire was used; menopause was defined as the reported cessation of periods, and surgical menopause as the disappearance of menstruation following a gynaecological operation. Although surgical and natural menopause similarly affected the slope of systolic pressure on age (Fig. 2, left panel), the former compared with the latter tended to be accompanied by a less pronounced upward shift of the relationship of diastolic pressure with age (Fig. 2, lower panel). It is possible that this was due to selective under-reporting of estrogen substitution in women having undergone surgical menopause, or to having included in the analysis one woman with hysterectomy only and 16 subjects in whom the exact nature of the gynaecological operation was unknown. However, at the time of the survey, estrogen replacement treatment following menopause was still regarded with scepticism by many Belgian women, while in Belgium, as in the Netherlands [4], hysterectomy is usually combined with oophorectomy. In previous studies, both an increased [7] and unchanged [8] blood pressure have been reported following oophorectomy.

The steeper slope of systolic pressure on age following menopause probably contributed to the increased pulse pressure observed in the present postmenopausal subjects (Table 1). The steeper increase with age in systolic pressure also suggests that following menopause the stiffness of the great arteries increases. This hypothesis is in agreement with a recent Dutch study [4], in which women were examined radiographically for calcified deposits in the abdominal aorta. After adjustment in the latter study for age and other cardiovascular risk indicators, women with natural menopause were found to have a three times greater risk of having atherosclerosis than premenopausal subjects, and women with surgical menopause a 5.5 greater risk.

Association in an epidemiological study does not imply causation. With this restriction in mind, several hypothetical mechanisms may be considered to explain the increase in blood pressure after menopause. For instance, the gain in weight, which in the present and in other [9, 12] studies accompanied menopause, may lead to hyperinsulinaemia. Insulin, within its physiological range, amy stimulate sodium reabsorption be the distal nephron without a change in the glomerular filtration rate or in the plasma concentration of aldosterone [14]. Hyperinsulinaemia may therefore be the common factor, also explaining the increased slope of diastolic pressure on body mass index and on the urinary sodium:potassium ratio (Fig. 3). Alternatively, the drop in the circulating sex steroids following menopause may affect the balance between various vasoactive hormones [16, 17]. Estrogen deficiency may influence the proliferation [18] and function of vascular smooth muscle cells, possibly by altering the electrolyte composition of the intra- [17] or extracellular [19, 20] environment. Finally, menopause through a redistribution of body sodium [19, 20] and the cessation of periods may lead to a rise in haemoglobin [8, 10] and in the count of red blood cells. The ensuing augmentation of blood viscosity may also be implicated in the rise in blood pressure with menopause.

Acknowledgements. This study was originally published in 1989 in the Journal of Human Hypertension 3:427–433 and is reproduced with permission from the publisher. The present survey would not have been possible without the collaboration of the population and General Practitioners. This work was supported by the Province of Limburg (Hasselt, Belgium), the municipalities Hechtel-Eksel and Lommel, the Belgian National Fund for Medical Research (Brussels, Belgium), the International Lead Zinc Research Organisation (Research Triangle Park, North Carolina USA), the Belgian Incentive Program *'Health Hazards'* (Science Policy Office, Prime Minister's Services, Brussels, Belgium) and Astra Pharmaceuticals Inc. (Brussels, Belgium). The filed work was co-ordinated by Mrs. S Van Hulle and conducted with the help from Mrs. L. Gijsbers, Mrs. A. Hermans, Mrs E. Jansen, Mrs. O. Palmans and Mrs. C Schraepen. Secretarial assistance was provided by Mrs. I. Tassens and Mrs. Y. Toremans.

References

1. Higano N, Robinson RW, Cohen WD (1963) Increased incidence of cardiovascular disease in castrated women: two-year follow-up studies. N Engl J Med 268:1123–1125
2. Weiss NS (1972) Premature menopause and aortoiliac occlusive disease. J Chron Dis 25:133–138
3. Colditz GA, Willett WC, Stampfer MJ, Rosner B, Speizer FE, Hennekens CH (1987) Menopause and the risk of coronary heart disease in women. N Engl J Med 316:1105–1110
4. Witteman JCM, Grobbee DE, Kok FJ, Hofman A, Valkenburg HA (1989) Increased risk of atherosclerosis in women after menopause. Br Med J 298:642–644
5. Kannel WB, Hjortland MC, McNamara PM, Gordon T (1976) Menopause and risk of cardiovascular disease: the Framingham Study. Ann Intern Med 85:447–452
6. Staessen J, Blupitt C, Fagard R, Joossens JV, Lijnen P, Amery A (1983) Four urinary cations and blood pressure: a population study in two Belgian towns. Am J Epidemiol 117:676–687
7. Weiss NS (1972) Relationship of menopause to serum cholesterol and arterial pressure: the United States Health Examination Survey of Adults. Am J Epidemiol 96:237–241
8. Hjörtland MC, McNamara PM, Kannel WB (1976) Some atherogenic concommitants of menopause: the Framingham Study. Am J Epidemiol 103:304–311
9. Lindquist O (1982) Intra-individual changes of blood pressure, serum lipids and body weight in relation to menstrual status : results from a prospective population study in Göteborg, Sweden. Prev Med 11:162–172
10. Lindquist O (1982) Influence of menopause on ischaemic heart disease and its risk factors and on bone mineral content. Acta Obstet Gynecol Scand Suppl 110:1–32
11. Lindquist O, Bengtsson C, Lapidus L (1985) Relationships between the menopause and risk factors for ischaemic heart disease. Acta Obstet Scand Suppl 130:43–47

12. Eferakeya AE, Imasuen JE (1986) Relationship of menopause to serum cholesterol and arterial blood pressure in some Nigerian women. Public Health 100:28–32
13. Kleinbaum DG, Kupper LL, Muller KE (1987) Applied regression analysis and other multivariable methods. PWS, Boston, pp 260–296
14. DeFronzo Ra, Cooke CR, Andres R, Falooha GR, Davis PJ (1975) The effect of insulin on renal handling of sodium, potassium, calcium, and phosphate in man. J Clin Invest 55:845–855
15. DeFronzo RA (1981) The effect of insulin on renal sodium metabolism. A review with clinical implications. Diabetologia 21:165–171
16. Sundsfjord JA, Aakvaag A (1972) Plasma renin activity, plasma renin substrate and urinary aldosterone excretion in the menstrual cycle in relation to the concentration of progesterone and estrogens in the plasma. Acta Endocrinol 71:519–525
17. M'Buyamba-Kabangu JR, Lijnen P, Fagard R, Groeseneken D, Koninckx P, Lissens W, Van Assche F, Amery A (1985) Erythrocyte concentrations and transmembrane fluxes of sodium and potassium and biochemical measurements during the menstrual cycle in normal women. Am J Obstet Gynecol 151:687–693
18. Fischer-Dzoga K, Wissler RW, Vesselinovitch D (1983) The effect of estradiol on the proliferation of rabbit aortic tissue culture cells induced by hyperlipemic serum. Exp Mol Pathol 39:355–363
19. Aitken JM, Lindsay R, Hart DM (1974) The redistribution of body sodium in women on longterm estrogen therapy. Cli Sci Mol Med 47:179–187
20. Hodgkinson A (1982) Plasma electrolyte concentrations in women and the effects of estrogen administration. Maturitas 4:247–256

Cardiovascular Disease in Women: Influence of Hormonal Replacement Therapy

Rogerio A. Lobo

Introduction

While the average age of menopause (approximately 51.3 years) has not changed for several centuries, life expectancy in the developed world has dramatically increased and now approaches 80 years. Fully one third of a woman's life is currently spent in an estrogen-deficient state. As the world's population increases, an increasing segment of the population is entering menopause or is already postmenopausal. In the United States, by the year 2015 it is estimated that 45 % of the population will be over age 45 [1].

Cardiovascular disease (CVD), specifically coronary artery disease (CAD), is the leading cause of death in older women [2]. In the United States, 500 000 women die annually from CVD and half of these are due to acute myocardial infarction. Forty percent of all coronary events in women are fatal [3]. Disability due to CVD is also substantial, with 36 % of women disabled by ischemic heart disease between the ages of 55 and 64 and 55 % in women over age 75. In the United States in 1991, the cost of CVD was estimated to be $117.4 billion (U.S. dollars) [4]. Fifty-eight percent of these health care costs are related to disease in women.

Therefore, CVD in women which has not received appreciable attention until recently in terms of teaching, research and public awareness, should move to the forefront of priorities in research and health care. A greater understanding of the etiology and prevention of CVD in women is imperative. This review will focus on the notion that estrogen deficiency is a major trigger for the acceleration of cardiovascular risk after menopause and that hormonal therapy is of substantial benefit.

Effects of Estrogen Deprivation

It appears clear that estrogen deprivation increases the risk of CVD in women. Data from the Framingham Study have been used to compare the incidence of CVD in men and women as they age. While the incidence is three times lower in women than in men prior to the menopause (3.1/1000 per year in women aged 45–49), it is approximately equal in men and women aged 75–79, being 53 and 50.4/1000 per year, respectively [5]. This trend also pertains to gender differences in mortality due to CVD.

While CVD only becomes more prevalent in later years following a natural menopause, premature cessation of ovarian function (prior to menopause) constitutes an additional risk [6, 7]. Premature menopause, occurring before age 35, was shown to increase the risk for myocardial infarction two- to threefold and premature oophorectomy (prior to age 35) increased the risk sevenfold [6]. What causes this increased risk?

When the possible reasons are examined for gender differences in the increase in CVD as a function of age, the most relevant finding appears to be that total cholesterol rises at an accelerated rate in postmenopausal women. While changes with age, weight, blood pressure and blood glucose are not thought to be substantially different in men and women, the rate of rise in total cholesterol after menopause is significantly different [8] (Table 1). This increase in total cholesterol is explained by increases in levels of low-density lipoprotein cholesterol (LDL-C).

In the Framingham cross-sectional study, high-density lipoprotein cholesterol (HDL-C) was not found to decrease after menopause although total cholesterol, LDL-C and very low density lipoprotein (VLDL) did increase. However, in a short-term longitudinal study [9], it was observed that after natural menopause, HDL-C did decrease with time. This is also in keeping with studies showing a decrease in HDL-C after the abrupt cessation of ovarian functions such as with oophorectomy or in some studies after the use of a gonadotropin-releasing hormone analog [10].

Much significance has been placed on changes in HDL-C, specifically on the benefits achieved by raising HDL-C with estrogen "replacement" therapy in postmenopausal women. This effect which is largely due to the increase in HDL_2-C with oral estrogen will be reviewed below. Nevertheless, the changes in HDL-C after a natural menopause may not be marked and HDL-C levels, for the most part, remain in the normal range. Curiously, in

Table 1. Framingham study: averages of some cardiovascular risk factors for men and women aged 30–59 years

	Blood Pressure (mmHg)				Serum		Blood	
	Systolic		Diastolic		Cholesterol (mg/dl)		Glucose (mg/dl)	
Age	Men	Women	Men	Women	Men	Women	Men	Women
30–34	125.2	116.7	79.3	73.5	218.0	198.0	80.0	78.1
35–39	127.6	119.6	81.6	76.0	223.8	204.8	79.2	79.7
40–44	131.1	125.6	84.0	79.7	228.6	219.2	81.5	80.6
45–49	130.9	133.9	84.2	83.2	229.7	230.4	84.7	82.4
50–54	135.6	144.7	85.7	87.5	229.9	247.4	84.9	84.1
55–59	140.7	151.5	85.3	88.0	229.2	257.1	84.1	86.8

From Kannel and Gordon (1987) [8]

the Pittsburgh study [9], there were no changes in HDL_2-C and no HDL-C changes with estrogen treatment. It is my view, therefore, that although HDL-C changes are important, the increases which occur with estrogen (the raising of "normal" levels by up to 15 %) may be viewed as pharmacologic and may not be as important as previously thought. Moreover, these alterations may merely be markers of other more important changes occurring in cholesterol transport. More data are clearly needed on the effects of estrogen deprivation and estrogen "replacement" on subspecies of LDL-C, oxidized forms of LDL-C and on lipoprotein(a), Lp(a). Recent data suggest that Lp(a) may rise after menopause and we have shown that Lp(a) is also lowered with estrogen [11].

Apart from the lipid hypothesis as reviewed briefly above, there is good reason to believe that there are direct arterial effects of estrogen. Therefore, the lack of arterial estrogen receptor activation in a state of estrogen deprivation may affect the endothelium in such a way that atherosclerotic plaque formation is accelerated and vascular tone is similarly compromised. These effects will be discussed more specifically below.

Cardioprotective Effects of Estrogens

Some of the confusion arising regarding estrogen use and cardiovascular function is because postmenopausal estrogen has been equated with the use of oral contraceptives. While the estrogen in oral contraceptives (ethinyl estradiol 30–50 μg) may exert some small cardiovascular risk, primarily on coagulation, this dose is at least 100 times greater than the dose used for postmenopausal replacement. Indeed estrogen replacement is cardioprotective.

At least 15 cohort (prospective) studies on postmenopausal estrogen use have shown there to be a significantly reduced risk of CVD when either fatal or nonfatal myocardial infarction was used as an end point (RR range, 0.3–0.7). Two recent meta-analyses have been carried out by Bush and Stampfer [12, 13] for the effect of estrogen on coronary heart disease risk and both have come to nearly identical conclusions. The calculated RR for all studies taken together was 0.56 (0.5–0.61) [13] and by including only those studies that were angiographic, prospective and internally controlled, the RR was 0.5 (0.43–0.56). For mortality specifically, the RR was also similar. This cardiovascular benefit has been demonstrated to occur in all age and socioeconomic groups and occurs even in women with high risk factors such as obesity and in women who smoke. In the United States, the data have been derived virtually exclusively with the use of conjugated equine estrogens (0.625 or 1.25 mg) and does not appear to have a dose response relationship. Mortality from stroke in one study [14] was also shown to be reduced by 40 %–50 % and here a small trend towards a dose response relationship was found. The United States National Health Survey Study also confirmed this finding recently. The effect of estrogen in reducing stroke mortality has not been found in all studies, but many investigators concur with this view.

Because of the high fatality rate attributable to ischemic heart disease, a RR of 0.5 translates into many lives saved among estrogen users. This has been estimated to be 5250 for every 100 000 estrogen users in the age range 50–75 years [15] (Table 2) or 333 lives annually (for ischemic heart disease and stroke) per 100 000 estrogen users in the age group 65–74 years. This change in mortality is greater than for any other disease potentially influenced by estrogen, including endometrial and breast cancer.

That postmenopausal estrogen use retards the progression of atherosclerosis is now becoming more widely accepted. Estrogen use has been associated with a reduction in angiographically defined coronary artery disease among women with chest pain as well as a reduction in the probalility of finding severe occlusive disease (odds ratio, 0.4) [16, 17]. Among women with greater than 70 % coronary artery occlusion, the 10 year survival was significantly greater (97 %) in estrogen users, and was only 65 % in nonusers of estrogen [18]. The benefit of estrogen also appeared to be greater when more severe disease (occlusion) was present.

The benefit of estrogen also appears to be related to duration of use. In the Leisure World Cohort Study [19], all-cause mortality was reduced by 40 % with 15 or more years of estrogen use. While this improvement in mortality was primarily due to a reduction in deaths due to CVD, other causes, including cancer, were also reduced.

The mechanisms for the cardioprotective effect of estrogen in postmenopausal women are not clear. Epidemiologic evidence has suggested that this effect is "substantially" mediated by the increase in HDL-C with the use of oral estrogen [12]. However, it is clear that there are other important effects of estrogen. The raising of HDL-C may be responsible for no more than 30 %–40 % of the ascribed benefit of estrogen "replacement" therapy. The

Table 2. Estimated changes in mortality induced by daily estrogen replacement therapy (0.625 mg) in women aged 50–75 years

Condition	Relative risk	Cumulative change in mortality/100 000
Osteoporotic fractures	0.4	– 563
Gallbladder disease	1.5	+ 2
Endometrial cancer	2.0	+ 63[a]
Breast cancer	1.1	+ 187
Ischemic heart disease	0.5	– 5250[b]

From Henderson et al. (1986) [15]
[a]Case fatality rate estimate at 0.05.
[b]Net change, – 5561; net percentage change, 41 %.

raising of normal HDL-C levels may be viewed as being a pharmacological, yet beneficial response. However, this change in HDL-C may merely be a marker of other changes in lipoprotein metabolism which includes reverse cholesterol transport.

A growing body of data supports the notion that the cardioprotective effects of estrogen are mediated directly by effects of estrogen on the arterial wall. Whether the mechanism is related primarily to direct changes in arterial tone or to changes in lipoprotein metabolism in the arterial wall is not clear and there is evidence for both mechanisms being operative. The uptake of LDL-C by the arterial wall has been shown to be enhanced by estrogen [20].

Studies in the macaque have shown that coronary atherosclerosis is significantly reduced in monkeys fed a high fat diet even when HDL-C has been reduced [21] (Fig. 1). This effect has been ascribed to the potent effects of ethinyl estradiol. In a postmenopausal macaque model, oophorectomized monkeys developed significant coronary atherosclerosis but were protected from this if they received nonoral estrogen "replacement" or estrogen with progesterone [22] (Fig. 2). With this nonoral hormonal regimen, HDL-C levels were not affected. When these monkeys were challenged with acetylcholine, the coronary arteries of the nontreated monkeys demonstrated a constriction response characteristic of endothelial damage due to atherosclerosis while the estrogen replaced monkeys did not [23] (Fig. 3). These and other data suggest that estrogen modulates the endothelium and causes the production of factors such as endothelial-derived relaxing factor or nitric oxide. Recent data have also confirmed that inhibition of nitric oxide with LLNA eliminates the increase in coronary blood flow induced by estrogen [24].

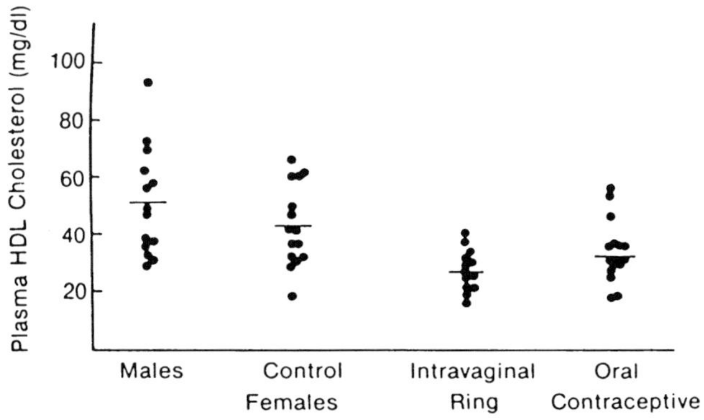

Fig. 1. Plasma high-density lipoprotein (HDL) cholesterol concentrations among four experimental groups. Females using intravaginal rings and oral contraceptives are not different ($p > 0.2$); both have lower plasma HDL cholesterol than males (> 0.02) and control females ($p > 0.02$). Males and controls females are not different ($p > 0.2$) From Adams et al. (1987) [21]

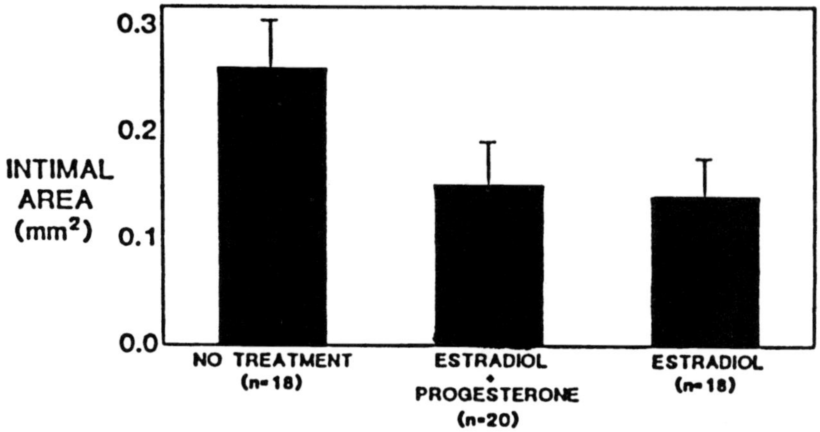

Fig. 2. Effect of ovariectomy and sex hormone replacement on extent of atherosclerosis expressed as mean intimal area + SEM. From Williams et al. (1990) [22]

Another mechanism which may be operative is a more favorable prostacyclin/thromboxane balance with estrogen. We have shown that prostacyclin production is reduced in postmenopausal uterine arteries [25] (Fig. 4). Other in vitro data [26] and our own preliminary prospective clinical data have shown that estrogen increases 6-keto-prostaglandin $F_{1\alpha}$ production. The effects of estrogen on endothelin production and action remains speculative

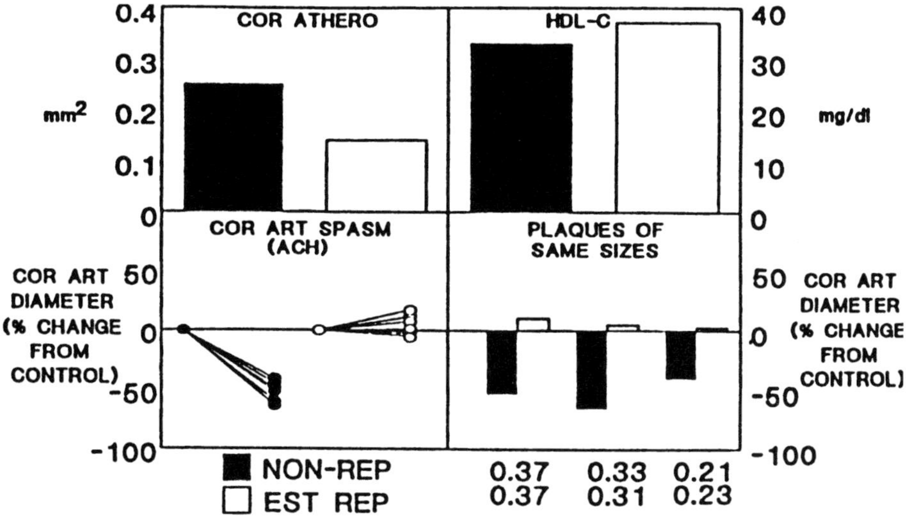

Fig. 3. Effect of estrogen replacement (*EST REP*) or no estrogen replacement (*NON REP*) on coronary artery plaque size (cross-sectional area in mm^2), plasma high-density lipoprotein cholesterol (*HDL-C*) concentrations and the response of coronary arteries to acetylcholine (*ACH*) injection. From Williams et al. (1991) [23]

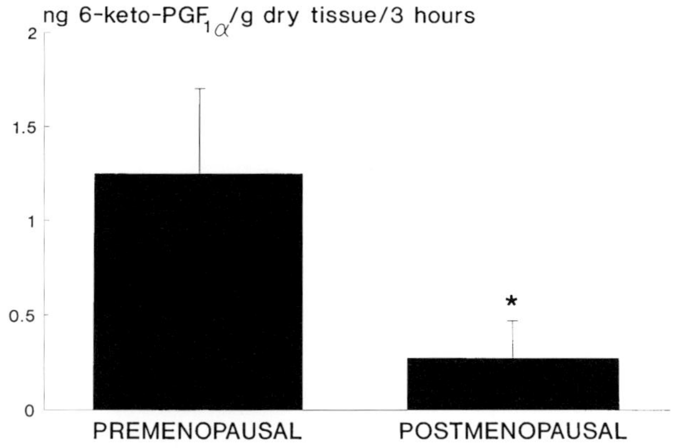

Fig. 4. Effect of 17β-estradiol on total steady state in vitro 6-keto-prostaglandin $F_{1\alpha}$ (*6-keto-PGF$_1$*) production by uterine arteries from pre- and postmenopausal women. From Steinleitner et al. (1989) [25]

at this time. Nevertheless, these findings taken together are compatible with human data showing that estrogen increases blood flow and decreases peripheral resistance. Uterine artery, aortic and carotid blood flow have been shown to increase with estrogen [27–29]. The reduction in the pulsatility index of carotid vessels with estrogen is depicted in (Fig. 5).

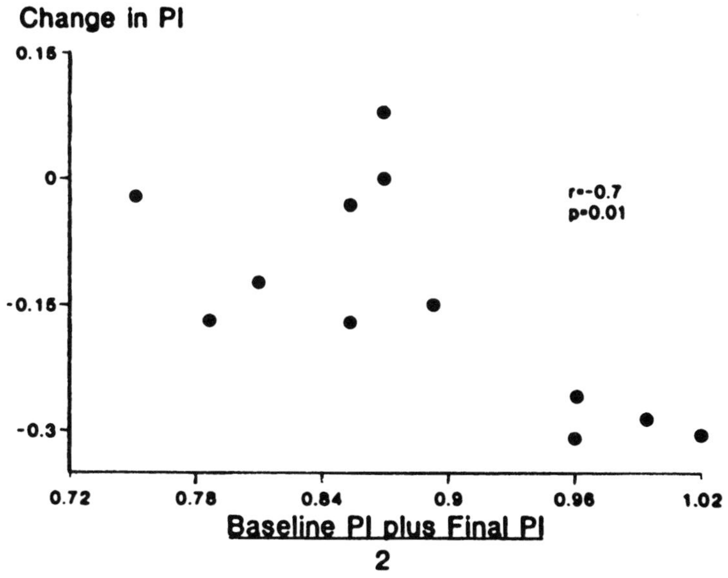

Fig. 5. Correlation between change in ponderal index (*PI*; between end of study and baseline) and mean of baseline and final PI values. From Gangar et al. (1991) [29]

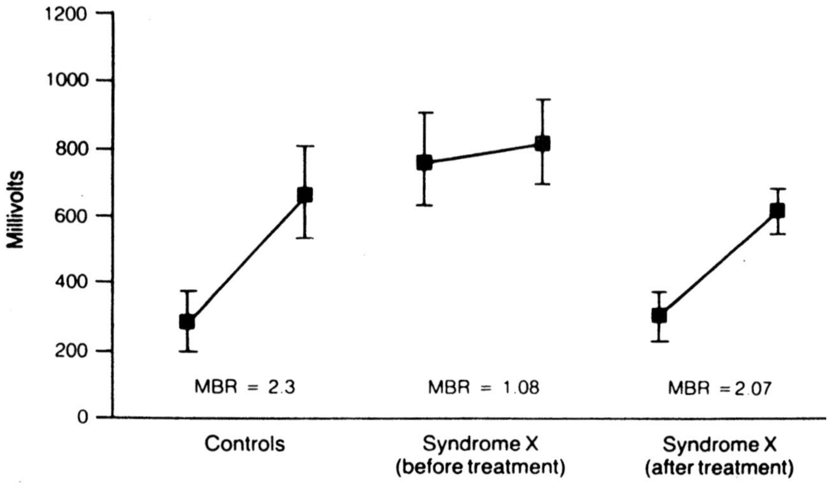

Fig. 6. Ratio of maximum to baseline flow of hyperemic response in women with syndrome X before and after treatment with 17β-estradiol compared with that of control subjects. From Sarrel et al. (1992) [30]

Although detailed human studies are lacking, recent work has suggested that estrogen mediates nitric oxide relase as well as having calcium antagonist activity. In women with chest pain and normal coronary arteries (syndrome X), the hyperemic response to occlusion in the forearm was restored after estrogen [30] (Fig. 6). Recently, sublingual estradiol was shown to improve exercise time and time to ST suppression in women with angina [31] (Fig. 7). The rapidity of some of these responses has led to the theory that estrogen works in a nongenomic way, possibly by antagonizing calcium channels. This attractive hypothesis is supported by several in vitro studies [32]. It is also conceivable that the effects of nitric oxide are also linked to inhibition of calcium channels.

Among many other potential cardioprotective effects of estrogen, two other deserve a brief discussion. Carbohydrate tolerance in postmenopausal women which was thought to be adversely affected (because of the equation of postmenopausal estrogen use to oral contraceptives), may be improved with estrogen. Also, cardiovascular reactivity to stress, which in animals is linked to accelerated atherosclerosis, is increased in postmenopausal women but is inhibited by estrogen.

Estrogen in vitro has been shown to increase insulin receptor binding [33]. In a cross-sectional study, postmenopausal user of estrogen were shown to have lower fasting insulin and glucose compared to nonusers [34]. Finally, we have shown that estrogen in moderate doses improved insulin sensitivity but that progestins and higher doses of oral estrogen may eliminate this effect [35]. More recent data from our group has suggested that this bimodal effect of estrogen is related to the oral route of administration.

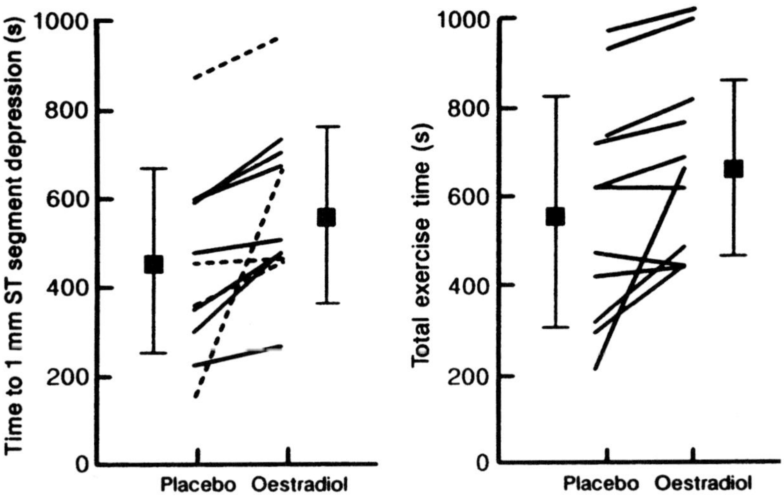

Fig. 7. Effect of estradiol-17β on time to 1 mm ST segment depression (*left*) and total exercise time (*right*). From Rosano et al. (1993) [31]

Transdermal estrogen which achieves fairly high levels of estrogen appeared to have a beneficial effect of improving insulin sensitivity.

Cardiovascular stress reactivity in postmenopausal women may be an important risk factor for CVD and atherosclerosis in particular. Compared to premenopausal women, postmenopausal women have increased blood pressure responses to evoked stress and increases in cortisol, ACTH and norepinephrine. These responses are blunted by estrogen but not by placebo [36].

Concerns of Blood Pressure, Coagulation and Lipids

Again, because of equating oral contraceptives to postmenopausal estrogen use, there has been a misconception about the role of estrogen on these parameters. Indeed, there is no real concern regarding blood pressure and coagulation changes and lipid and lipoprotein profiles are favorable with estrogen use. These will be reviewed briefly below.

Blood Pressure

Natural estrogens either impart no change in blood pressure or lower it in the majority of both normotensive and hypertensive women so treated. In approximately 5 % of postmenopausal women, an idiosyncratic elevation of blood pressure has been observed with the use of conjugated equine estro-

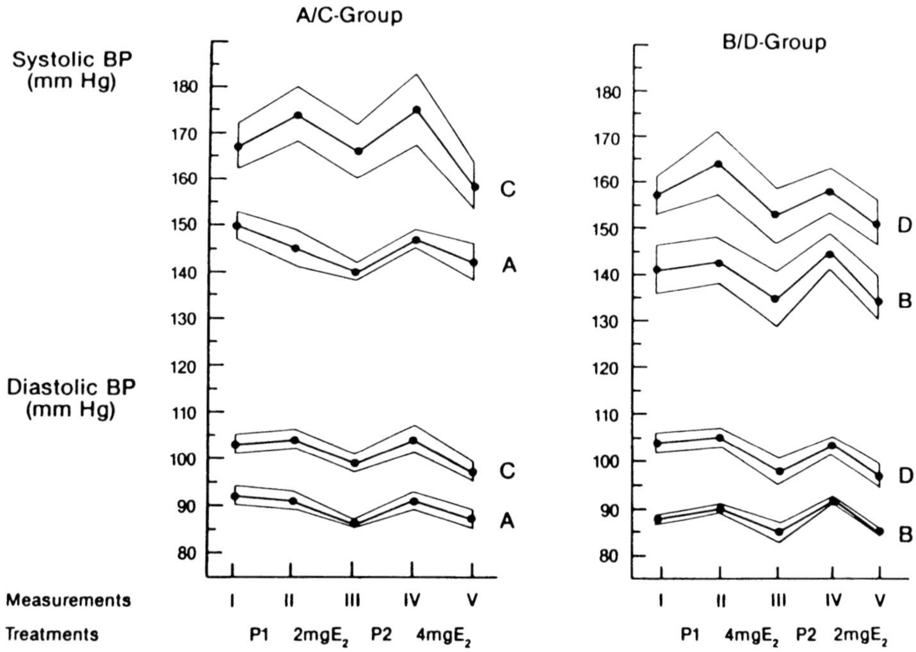

Fig. 8. The effect of micronized estradiol (E_2) on diastolic and systolic blood pressure in normotensive (*A* and *B* groups) and hypertensive (*C* and *D* groups) women. Shown are mean values ± SEM for blood pressure in supine position. *P*, placebo. From Luotola (1983)[38]

gens [37]. However, the occurrence of sensitivity to this estrogen is rare and does not contraindicate other forms of estrogen "replacement". Figure 8 illustrates the lowering of blood pressure in both hypertensive and normotensive women receiving two doses of micronized estradiol [38]. These changes are compatible with data showing a vasodilatory effect of estrogen resulting in increased blood flow. More recent findings have found in a 2-year placebo controlled longitudinal study that while diastolic blood pressure increased with placebo, blood pressure was not affected by oral or transdermal estradiol [39]. While oral estradiol increased renin substrate while transdermal did not, there was no correlation with blood pressure changes.

Coagulation

Although the ethinyl estradiol content of OCs has been implicated in thromboembolic risk because of increases in levels of procoagulant factors produced by the liver, this does not occur with natural estrogen "replacement". Figure 9 shows a similar effect of oral estrone sulfate and placebo on Factor

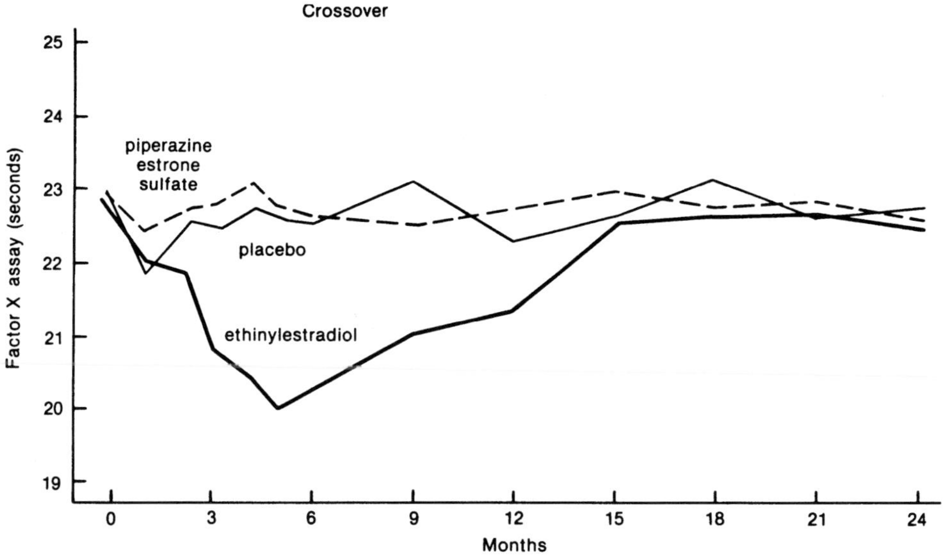

Fig. 9. Factor X assays during initial 6-month comparative trial and during the following 18 months after crossover to piperazine estrone sulfate (mg/day). From Aylward et al. (1977) [40]

X activity, while 30 µg 3-methyl ether of ethinyl estradiol (mestranol) has a potentially deleterious effect [40]. Conjugated equine estrogens administered with and without progestin, in doses of 0.625 and 1.25 mg daily, have been shown not to have a deleterious effect on procoagulant factors [41, 42]. A recent case control study has confirmed that there is no increased risk of thromboembolic phenomena occurring with estrogen "replacement" [43]. In the editorial accompanying this report [44] it was suggested that while the risk of coagulopathy in "normal" postmenopausal women is not increased, there are women who are more susceptible to the effects of estrogen. These women are diffcult to identify by routine blood tests. In patients with a history of coagulation problems associated with exposure to increased levels of estrogen (pregnancy, oral contraceptives) or even with routine "replacement" therapy, great caution should be exercised. In this setting "physiologic" replacement with transdermal estradiol might be considered, thus, by passing the hepatic "first passage" effect. Monitoring of serum estradiol levels would assure that an acceptable range of estrogen is achieved.

Lipids and Lipoproteins

The effects of estrogen on lipids and lipoproteins are not considered to be a risk factor, but in fact the reverse is the case. These effects have been viewed to be the primary cardioprotective feature of estrogen "replacement".

Details of this interaction have been reviewed recently [45]. Figure 10 depicts a summary of the changes expected with oral estrogen use (the equivalent of 0.625 mg conjugated equine estrogens). The principal cardioprotective benefit is thought to be related to the increase in HDL-C (specifically in HDL_2-C) and the lowering of LDL-C which is more variable.

The only potential cause for concern with oral estrogen is hypertriglyceridemia. This change is highly variable, with some women showing very small changes with oral estrogen and others having a dramatic increase. Indeed in these rare patients, oral estrogen may not be the preferable route of administration. The changes in all lipoproteins are thought to be dose dependent, but it has been suggested that by keeping doses of conjugated euqine estrogens to 0.625 mg, total triglycerides and the triglyceride content of lipoproteins will be kept to a low percentage [46]. While it is generally thought that there is an important dose response increase in HDL-C with oral estrogen, a saturation effect does occur and near maximum benefit is thought to be achieved with doses of 0.625 mg conjugated equine estrogens [45, 46].

Nonoral forms of estrogen "replacement" do not achieve the same degree of stimulation of HDL-C and HDL_2-C, but sufficient doses of estrogen, prescribed for at least 6 months, have resulted in significant elevations in HDL-C and a lowering of the C to HDL ratio [47] (Fig. 11). With nonoral routes of administration, as illustrated in this figure, triglycerides levels are not increased.

Most recently, data have emerged that estrogen may exhibit antioxidant activity. In that oxidation of LDL is implicated in atherogenesis, this may be

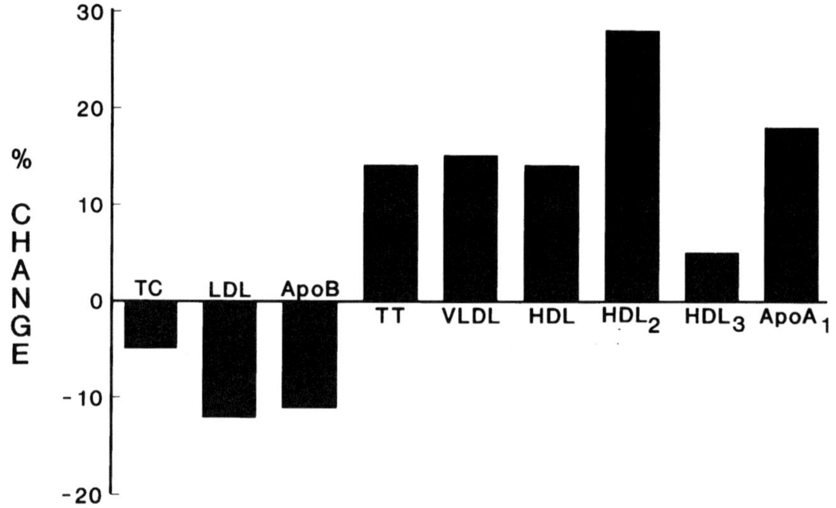

Fig. 10. Percent age changes in lipids and lipoproteins with the use of oral estrogen (equivalent to 0.625 mg for at least 3 months). *TC*, total cholesterol; *TT* total triglcycerides; *LDL*, low-density lipoprotein; *Apo*, apoprotein; *VLDL*, very low density lipoprotein; *HDL*, high-density lipoprotein. From Lobo (1991) [45]

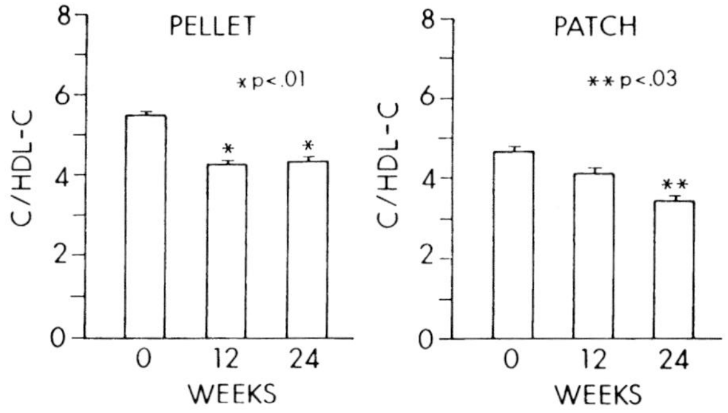

Fig. 11. Mean (± SEM) serum total cholesterol (*C*) to high-density lipoprotein cholesterol (*HDL-C*) ratio before and during 12 and 24 weeks of subdermal (pellet; left) and transdermal (patch; right) estradiol treatment. The significance of difference in the comparison of the C to HDL-C ratios at 12 and 24 weeks with the baseline value is represented as $*p<0.01$ and $**p<0.03$. From Stancyzk et al. (1988) [47]

an important beneficial effect of estrogen. Equine estrogens in vitro have been shown to exhibit greater activity than estradiol [48].

Impact of Progestins

All the epidemiologic data for postmenopausal women reviewed above pertain to the cardiovascular effects of estrogen alone and have not as yet been analyzed for the addition of progestins. On a theoretical basis, progestins may have a negative impact on cardiovascular function and can also lead to mood changes and patient discomfort. Therefore, the addition of a progestin is only indicated in women with a uterus, where endometrial protection is needed.

Progestins have a number of potential adverse effects on the cardiovascular system although there are as yet no published epidemiological data. Some data are, nevertheless, of concern. In one study of mentally retarded women (aged 35–51 years) treated with a continuous synthetic progestin, lynoestrenol, to induce amenorrhea, eight of 19 (42 %) showed evidence of arterial disease at autopsy compared with only one of 15 (7 %) untreated women [49]. Several factors might account for the detrimental effects of progestin on cardiovascular function. The first is the lipid hypothesis which postulates a reduction in HDL-C and HDL_2-C during progestin exposure [45]. Second, the potential downregulation of estrogen receptors in all tissues including coronary vessels. Three, the inhibition of endothelial prostacyclin. Four, a decrease or attenuation is estrogen mediated blood flow. Five, a dose related progestational effect adversely influencing carbohydrate tolerance. Finally, a change in the quality of life because mood disturbances may occur or increase when receiving progestins.

Most progestin mediated effects on lipoproteins are dose and duration related. High doses of progestins are likely to cause the following changes: a reduction in HDL-C and even an increase in LDL-C, although triglycerides are usually lowered. However, the balance or ratio between the estrogen and progestin doses is extremely important. A high estrogen dose may overcome any harmful progestin effects. The greater the progestin's androgenic potency, the greater is its propensity for adverse metabolic effects.

The inhibition of HDL-C is largely dose related. However, even 10 mg medroxyprogesterone acetate, a 17-hydroxyprogesterone derivative, attenuates HDL-C by about 8% and HDL_2-C by about 17%. Sherwin [49] showed that the beneficial effects of conjugated equine estrogens (0.625–1.25 mg) on HDL-C and LDL-C may be attenuated by the addition of as little as 5 mg medroxyprogesterone acetate. The overall effects of various progestins on lipoproteins [45] may be found in Table 3.

Even natural progesterone which is more metabolically inert has been shown to completely abolish the estrogen induced changes in prostacyclin in human umbilical arteries in vitro [26]. Similarly, several studies have shown that progestins decrease uterine blood flow. Taken together, these data suggest that all progestins influence various parameters of cardiovascular function to some extent. Interestingly, however, in the monkey data reviewed above (Fig. 2), physiologic levels of progesterone, administered systemically, did not attenuate the beneficial effects of estrogen in reducing coronary atherosclerosis. Clearly, the type of progestin, its dose as well as the route of administration are all extremely important in this interaction. It appears, therefore, that although progestins have potentially adverse effects on cardiovascular function, if it is administered in lower doses and using a more metabolically inert progestin, preferably progesterone itself, that these effects can be minimized or eliminated. A recent small Swedish study found the protective effect of estradiol valerate on the incidence of myocardial infarction to be similar with and without an added progestin (levonorgestrel) [50].

Table 3. Percentage change in lipoproteins with various progestins

	Micronized P (200 mg)	MPA (5 mg)	MPA (10 mg)	NET (1 ng)	dl–NG (0.15)	(0.25)
HDL	–2	–6	–6%	–10	–14	–18%
HDL_2	0	–11	–19%	–27	–23	–25
HDL_3	0	0	–2%	–1%	0	–8
LDL	0	+3	+7%	+10%	+6	+1
Apo A_1	+1	–5	–11%	–11%	–15	–15
Apo B	0	0	+3%	+10%	+8	+10

HDL, high–density lipoprotein; LDL, low–density lipoprotein; Apo, apoprotein. Micronized P, micronized progesterone; MPA, medroxyprogesterone acetate; NET, norethindrone; dl–NG, norgestrel, during sequential administration compared with the effects of unopposed estrogen.

An International Consensus Statement

In December, 1993, an International Consensus Meeting was convened to discuss the impact of hormonal therapy and CVD [51]. In essence, a consensus was reached that although prospective randomized studies would be beneficial, that there was substantial evidence supporting a role of estrogen in the prevention of CVD as well as its having a benefit in women with established disease. A majority opinion was that certain types and doses of progestins used for hormonal replacement were likely to attenuate the benefits of estrogen alone.

Dosage Regimens for Hormonal Replacement

Most clinicians currently favor daily estrogen administration although it is also routine to administer estrogen for 25 days each month. If required, progestins are administered for 10–14 days, either on a calendar basis if estrogen is prescribed daily, or on the last 10–14 days of a sequential 25 day regimen. A very popular regimen is "continuous combined" hormonal therapy where both estrogen and progestin are taken daily. While this was originally prescribed for each day of the year, now some clinicians are suggesting that it be taken for 5 days out of the week or for 25 days each month.

Because of potential deleterious effects of the progestins, my preference is to administer progestins sequentially for 10 days per cycle. Suitable progestins include medroxyprogesterone acetate (5 mg), norethindrone (1 mg) and 200 mg micronized progesterone. Even lower doses may be prescribed if side effects are encountered. While these and larger doses are known to cause secretory transformation of the endometrium, this occurrence is probably not necessary to avoid endometrial hyperplasia.

The occurrence of amenorrhea due to an atrophic endometrium may be achieved in women receiving continuous combined therapy. Although bleeding (spotting) may occur in the first few months, amenorrhea usually ensues. Depending on the combination, a continuous combined regimen may adversely affect the lipid profile. However, the magnitude of these changes and its significance has varied considerably between various studies because of marked differences in patient population and study design. Because of the unknown long-term cardiovascular effects of continuous progestogen exposure, it is my preference not to use this regimen as a first line regimen. However, on balance, if an adequate amount of estrogen is used, the progestogen effect is likely to be minimized.

If treatment with a progestogen is to be successful, the biochemical processes which cause hyperplasia must be reduced or blocked and mitotic activity diminished. It is unnecessary to induce a full range of secretory changes with large progestin doses. These larger doses generally lead to an increased amount of withdrawal bleeding. Prevention of hyperplasia necessitates a reduction in mitotic activity. This, and a reduction in bleeding, should be the principal aim of an effective regimen. With this approach, it is estimated that the maximal inhibitory effect on cardiovascular function (including arterial as well as lipoprotein effects) would be a 15 % reduction in the benefit for the 10 days of exposure [52]. This is not likely to affect RR estimates of the cardioprotective effects of hormonal replacement. Nevertheless, it is important to reiterate that only in women with a uterus is any progestin therapy indicated [53].

References

1. U.S. Senate Special Committee on Aging (1988) Aging america: trends and projections. United States Department of Health and Human Services, Washington
2. Sempos CT, Cleeman JI, Carroll MD et al. (1993) Prevalence of high blood cholesterol among U.S. adults: an update based on guidelines from the Second Report of the National Cholesterol Education Programm Adult Treatment Panel. JAMA 269:3009
3. Kannel WB, Abbott RD (1987) Incidence and prognosis of myocardial infarction in women: the Framingham study. In: Eaker ED, Packard B, Wenger NK, Clarkson TB, Tyroler HA (eds). Coronary heart disease in women. National Heart, Lung, and Blood Institute, National Institutes of Health, Bethesda
4. American Heart Association (1993) 1993 heart and stroke facts statistics. American Heart Association, Dallas
5. Kannel WB, Hjortland MC, McNamara PM et al. (1976) Menopause and the risk of cardiovascular disease: the Framingham study. Ann Intern Med 85:447
6. Rosenberg L, Hennekens CH, Rosner B et al. (1981) Early menopause and the risk of myocardial infarction. Am J Obstet Gynecol 139:47
7. Centerwall BS (1981) Premenopausal hysterectomy and cardiovascular disease. Am J Obstet Gynecol 139:58
8. Kannel WB, Gordon T (1987) Cardiovascular effects of the menopause. In: Mishell DR Jr (ed). Menopause: physiology and pharmacology. Year Book Medical, Chicago, p 91
9. Matthews KA, Meilahn E, Kuller LH, Kelsey SF, Caggiula AW, Wing RR (1989) Menopause and risk factors for coronary heart disease. N Engl J Med 321:641
10. Jensen J, Nilas L, Christiansen C (1990) Influence of menopause on serum lipids and lipoproteins. Maturitas 12:321
11. Lobo RA, Notelvitz M, Bernstein L, Khan FY, Ross RK, Paul WL (1992) Lp(a) lipoprotein: relationship to cardivascular disease risk factors, exercise, and estrogen. Am J Obstet Gynecol 166:1182
12. Bush RL (1990) Noncontraceptive estrogen use and risk of cardiovascular disease: an overview and critique of the literature. In: Korenman SG (ed). The menopause. Biological and clinical consequences of ovarian failure: evolution and management. Serono Symposium, Norwell, Massachusetts, p 211
13. Stampfer MJ, Willett WC, Colditz GA, Speizer FE, Hennekens CH (1990) Past use of oral contraceptives and cardiovascular disease: a meta-analysis in the context of the Nurses' Health Study. Am J Obstet Gynecol 163:285
14. Paganini-Hill A, Ross RK, Henderson BE (1988) Postmenopausal oestrogen treatment and stroke: prospective study. Br Med J 297:519

15. Henderson BE, Ross RK, Paganini-Hill A, Mack TM (1986) Estrogen use and cardiovascular disease. Am J Obstet Gynecol 154:1181
16. Sullivan JM, Vander Zwaag R, Lemp GF et al. (1988) Postmenopausal estrogen use and coronary atherosclerosis. Ann Intern Med 108:358
17. Gruchow HW, Anderson AJ, Barboriak JJ, Sobocinski KA (1988) Postemenopausal use of estrogen and occlusion of coronary arteries. Am Heart J 115:954
18. Sullivan JM, Vander Zwaag R, Hughes JP et al. (1990) Estrogen replacement and coronary artery disease. Arch Intern Med 150:2557
19. Henderson BE, Paganini-Hill A, Ross RK (1991) Decreased mortality in users of estrogen replacement therapy. Arch Intern Med 151:75
20. Wagner JD, Clarkson TB, Adams MR, Schwenke DC (1991) The effects of oral contraceptives on coronary artery LDL metabolism in female cynomolgus monkeys. Circulation 84[Suppl II]:II–602
21. Adams MR, Clarkson TB, Koritnik DR et al. (1987) Contraceptives, steroids and coronary artery atherosclerosis in cynomolgus macaques. Fertil Steril 47:1010
22. Williams JK, Adams MR, Klopfenstein HS (1990) Estrogen modulates responses of atherosclerotic coronary arteries. Circulation 81:1680
23. Williams JR, Adams MR, Herrington DM, Clarkson TB (1991) The effects of short-term estrogen treatment on vascular responses of coronary arteries. Circulation 84[Suppl II]:II–272
24. Lang U, Baker RS, Fisher BK, Yang D, Clark KE (1993) Estrogen increases coronary blood flow and is antagonized by inhibitors of nitric oxide (abstr no P353). Presented at the 40th annual meeting of the Society For Gynecologic Investigation, March 31–April 3, 1993, Toronto, Ontario
25. Steinleitner A, Stanczyk FZ, Levin JH et al. (1989) Decreased in vitro production of 6-keto-prostaglandin $F_{1\alpha}$ by uterine arteries from postmenopausal women. Am J Obstet Gynecol 161:1677
26. Makila UM, Wahlberg L, Vlinikka L, Ylikorkala O (1982) Regulation of prostacyclin and thromboxane production by human umbilical vessels. The effect of estradiol and progesterone in a superfusion model. Prostaglandins Leukot Med 8:115
27. Bourne T, Hillard TC, Whitehead MI, Crook D, Campbell S (1990) Estrogen, arterial status, and postmenopausal women. Lancet 335:1470
28. Pines A, Fisman EZ, Levo Y et al. (1991) The effects of hormone replacement therapy in normal postmenopausal women: measurement of Doppler-derived parameters of aortic flow. Am J Obstet Gynecol 64:806
29. Gangar KF, Vyas S, Whitehead M, Crook D, Meire H, Campbell S (1991) Pulsatility index in internal carotid artery in relation to transdermal oestradiol and time since menopause. Lancet 338:839
30. Sarrel PM, Lindsay D, Rosano GMC, Poole-Wilson PA (1992) Angina and normal coronary arteries in women: gynecologic findings. Am J Obstet Gynecol 167:467
31. Rosano GMC, Sarrel PM, Poole-Wilson P, Collins P (1993) Beneficial effect of estrogen on exercise-induced myocardial ischaemia in women with coronary artery disease. Lancet 342:133
32. Collins P, Rosano GMC, Jiang C, Lindsay D, Sarrel PM, Poole-Wilson PA (1993) Cardiovascular protection by estrogen – calcium antagonist effect? Lancet 341:1264
33. Ballejo G, Saleem TH, Khan-Dawood FS et al. (1983) The effect of sex steroids on insulin binding by target tissues in the rat. Contraception 28:413
34. Barrett-Connor E, Laakso M (1990) Ischemic heart disease risk in postmenopausal women. Effects of estrogen use on glucose and insulin levels. Arteriosclerosis 10:531
35. Lindheim SR, Presser SC, Ditkoff EC, Vijod MA, Stanczyk FZ, Lobo RA (1993) A possible bimodal effect of estrogen on insulin sensitivity in postmenopausal women and the attenuating effect of added progestin. Fertil Steril 60:664

36. Lindheim SR, Legro RS, Bernstein L et al. (1992) Behavioral stress responses in premenopausal and postmenopausal women and the effects of estrogen. Am J Obstet Gynecol 167:1831
37. Mashchak CA, Lobo RA (1985) Estrogen replacement therapy and hypertension. J Repro Med 30 [Suppl 10]:805
38. Luotola H (1983) Blood pressure and hemodynamics in postmenopausal women during estradiol-17β substitution. Ann Clin Res 15:1
39. Hassager C, Riis BJ, Strom V, Guyene TT, Christiansen C (1987) The long-term effect of oral and percutaneous estradiol on plasma renin substrate and blood pressure. Circulation 76:753
40. Aylward M, Maddock J, Lewis PA, Rees PL (1977) Estrogen replacement therapy and blood clotting. Curr Med Res Opin 4 [Suppl 3]:83
41. Notelovitz M, Ware M (1982) Coagulation risks with postmenopausal estrogen therapy. In: Studd J (ed) Progress in obstetrics and gynecology, vol 2. Churchill Livingstone, Edinburgh
42. Notelovitz M, Kitchens C, Ware MD et al. (1983) Combination estrogen and progestogen replacement therapy does not adversely affect coagulation. Obstet Gynecol 62:596
43. Devor M, Barrett-Connor E, Renvall M, Feigal D Jr, Ramsdell J (1992) Estrogen replacement therapy and the risk of venous thrombosis. Am J Med 92:275
44. Lobo RA (1992) Estrogen and the risk of coagulopathy. Am J Med 92:283
45. Lobo RA (1991) Effects of hormonal replacement on lipids and lipoproteins in postmenopausal women. J Clin Endocrinol Metab 73:925
46. Walsh BW, Schiff I, Rosner B, Greenberg L, Ravnikar V, Sacks FM (1991) Effects of postmenopausal estrogen replacement on the concentrations and metabolism of plasma lipoproteins. N Engl J Med 325:1196
47. Stanczyk FZ, Shoupe D, Nunez V, Macias-Gonzales P, Vijod MA, Lobo RA (1988) A randomized comparison of nonoral estradiol delivery in postmenopausal women. Am J Obstet Gynecol 159:1540
48. Subbiah MTR, Kessel B, Agrawal M, Rajan R, Abplanalp W, Rymaszewski Z (1993) Antioxidant potential of specific estrogens on lipid peroxidation. J Clin Endocrinol Metab 77:1095
49. Huovinen K, Autio S, Kaprio J (1988) Peroral lynestrenol and arterial disease in mentally retarded women. A case-control study based on autopsy findings. Acta Obstet Gynecol Scand 67:211
50. Falkeborn M, Persson I, Adami H-O et al. (1992) The risk of acute myocardial infarction after oestrogen and oestrogen-progestogen replacement. Br J Obstet Gynecol 99:821
51. Lobo RA, Speroff L (1994) International Consensus conference on postmenopausal hormone therapy and the cardiovascular system. Fertil Steril (in press)
52. Moyer DL, de Lignieres B, Drigues P, Pez JP (1993) Prevention of endometrial hyperplasia by progesterone during long-term estradiol replacement: influence of bleeding pattern and secretory changes. Fertil Steril 59:992
53. Lobo RA (1991) Which progestogen? What dosage? In: Proceedings of the International Novo Nordisk Symposium on cardiovascular effects of hormone replacement therapy. Copenhagen, February 1–2, 1991, Novo Nordisk A/S, p 97

Hormone Replacement Therapy in Hypertensive, Postmenopausal Women: Role of the Gynecologist

Karen Bradshaw

Postmenopausal women represent the largest category of women who are at risk for hypertension and coronary heart disease (CHD). The risk for CHD is not only due to the rise in lipid risk factors with age, but also because of the rise of other risk factors, most notably hypertension and diabetes with age. After menopause, the incidence of hypertension, cardiovascular disease and cardiovascular mortality increases progressively in women relative to men leading to an eventual equal incidence in both sexes. Most untreated women with hypertension will develop further increases in their arterial pressure with time. The most frequent cause of death among U.S. women is cardiovascular disease leading to approximately 250 000 deaths per year. This is approximately double the cancer mortality rate in women and six times that for breast cancer (44 000 deaths in 1992).

From actuarial data and also from experience in the era prior to effective therapy, it has been documented that untreated hypertension is associated with a shortening of life by 10–20 years, usually related to an acceleration of the atherosclerotic process, with the rate of acceleration in part related to the severity of the hypertension. The most common cause of premature death is heart disease, with stroke and renal failure as other frequent end stage disorders of chronic hypertension.

The effect of hypertension on the heart is related to cardiac compensation for the excessive workload imposed by increased systemic pressure. This excess workload is initially sustained by concentric left ventricular hypertrophy, characterized by an increase in wall thickness. Ultimately, the function of this chamber deteriorates, the cavity dilates, and the symptoms and signs of heart failure appear. Angina pectoris may also occur because of the combination of accelerated coronary arterial disease and increased myocardial oxygen requirements as a consequence of the increased myocardial mass.

On physical examination the heart is enlarged and has a prominent left ventricular impulse. The sound of aortic closure is accentuated, and there may be a faint murmur of aortic regurgitation. Presystolic (atrial, fourth) heart sounds appear frequently in hypertensive heart disease, and a summation gallop rhythm (ventricular, third heart sound) is sometimes present. Electrocardiogram (ECG) changes of left ventricular hypertrophy are common; evidence of ischemia or infarction may be observed late in the disease. The majority for deaths due to hypertension result from myocardial infarction or congestive heart failure.

Assessment of Postmenopausal Woman

The initial assessment of a postmenopausal woman in determining her risk for CHD is careful history and physical examination aimed at identifying all potential risk factors. The history should include questions concerning chest pain and exercise habits. Often overlooked, but an important risk factor is a family history of CHD and age of onset. In evaluating hypertension, testing should be directed at uncovering correctable secondary forms of hypertension such as fever, thyroid disease, valvular disease, chronic renal disease, or adrenocortical hyperfunction. The physician should also establish a pretreatment baseline, assess other risk factors such as diet, stress, medications, and assess compliance as a guide to type of therapy.

Few symptoms of elevated arterial pressure exist other than occipital headaches (more commonly present in the morning), dizziness, palpitations, easy fatigue ability. A general physical examination is done to search for systemic disease or funduscopic findings consistent with severe hypertension. Blood pressure and pulses are taken in the upper and lower extremities in supine and standing positions. A battery of automated tests can help in evaluating for a variety of disorders. Blood urea nitrogen (BUN), creatinine, potassium, blood glucose, uric acid, cholesterol and triglycerides, ECG, and chest X-ray are also important.

A 24-h dietary recall of dietary intake is useful as the first step in CHD prevention is maximization of dietary therapy to reduce dietary cholesterol. Reduction of saturated fatty acids, found mainly in animal fat, dairy fat, and hidden fats in products such as baked goods. Sources of dietary cholesterol including egg yolks, organ meats, as well as any animal product are targeted for reduction as well. The last major area in dietary modification for high cholesterol levels is total calories and body weight. Cross-sectional studies demonstrate that excess body weight raises total cholesterol and low-density lipoprotein (LDL) cholesterol levels in women and in men. The effects of body weight on raising total and LDL levels is seen most dramatically in young men, but is also present in older women. In addition to total cholesterol and LDL effects, excess body weight lowers high-density lipoprotein (HDL) cholesterol levels. The effects of body weight on HDL levels are seen in both sexes and at all ages. Since HDL cholesterol is a significant predictor of CHD, the clinical significance of excess body weight in producing low HDL levels should not be underestimated. In addition, there is evidence that peri-menopausal women are particularly susceptible to gaining weight during menopause which further compounds this problem.

Cardioprotective Effects of Estrogens

After an adequate trial of dietary therapy, the next approach is hormonal replacement therapy (HRT). HRT has salutary effects on serum lipids, with lowering of total cholesterol and LDL cholesterol, as well as slight increase in HDL. Other well known advantages of HRT besides lipid lowering include preventing osteoporosis, promotion of vaginal lubrication with the prevention of genito-urinary atrophy, and amelioration of hot flashes. Epidemiologic evidence also suggests that HRT may half the risk of CHD. The lowering of LDL cholesterol levels appears to be non-linear and on the current suggested replacement dose of 0.625 mg conjugated estrogens a day, a significant LDL reduction of 10–60 mg/dl is typically seen. However, if the estrogen dose is increased, significant rises in serum triglycerides result.

As cardiovascular disease is the major cause of death in the developed world, any influence that estrogen replacement therapy has in reducing the risk of this disease is of major importance in the overall risk-benefit equation. In the United States some 42.5 % of deaths among women over the age of 50 years are due to cardiovascular disease. By using a mathematical model to study the overall effects of estrogen therapy, it can be shown that more lives can be saved from the reduction in cardiovascular disease with estrogen use than from the reduction in death, from osteoporosis or any other disease state affected by estrogen.

Henderson et al. [1] computed the effect on mortality rate, to the age of 75 years, of 0.625 mg/day of conjugated estrogens given at 50 years of age to 100 000 representative U.S. women. The results are shown in Table 1. Clearly, the benefits in terms of reduced mortality associated with osteoporotic fractures and ischemic heart disease outweigh the risk of endometrial and breast cancer.

Table 1. Effect on mortality rate to the age of 75 years of 0.625 mg conjugated estrogens day given at 50 years of age to 100 000 U.S. women

Condition	Relative risk	Cumulative change in mortality per 100 000
Osteoporotic fractures	0.4	-563
Gallbladder disease	1.5	+2
Endometrial cancer	2.0	+63
Breast cancer	1.1	+187
Ischemic heart disease	0.5	-5250
Net change		-5561
Net % change		-41 %

Adapted from Henderson et al. [1]

Evidence from animal and autopsy studies indicates that exogenous estrogens inhibit the development of atherosclerotic coronary artery lesions. This is supported by coronary angiographic studies, where lower levels of coronary artery occlusion are seen in women treated with exogenous estrogens than in untreated women. Large case-control and prospective cohort studies have shown that estrogen reduces the risk of coronary heart disease and myocardial infarction in postmenopausal women. Meta-analysis of the relevant studies has shown a 45 % decrease in the risk of cardiovascular disease in women who have received estrogen replacement therapy after menopause.

Although it is clear that the estrogen-mediated changes in total cholesterol, HDL cholesterol, and LDL cholesterol are important factors in delineating the cardioprotective effects of estrogen (J.D. Litwin and J.S. Lippman, unpublished data), there is mounting evidence that estrogen has a beneficial effect on the cardiovascular system that is independent of its lipoprotein effects. Estrogen decrease LDL cholesterol and increase HDL cholesterol by mechanisms that include the possible induction of LDL receptors and the destruction of hepatic lipase, which degrades HDL cholesterol. However, estrogen also appears to have a direct beneficial effect on vessel wall physiology.

Estrogen receptors have been found in cells from disparate areas such as vagina, vulva, cervix, uterus, endometrium, bladder, breast, skin, bone, arteries, heart, liver, and brain. Receptors also have been demonstrated in the walls of blood vessels of various primates including man and it has been suggested that there may be a direct effect of estrogen in the inhibition of atheromatous plaque formation. Consistent with this hypothesis is the fact that estrogen reduces the formation of thromboxane. There is reduced smooth muscle proliferation and an associated decreased uptake of cholesterol. Other direct effects on the blood vessel wall (at the level of the arterial intima) have been demonstrated, including alterations in collagen and elastin formation, as well as changes in prostacyclin production.

The hypothesis that the cardioprotective mechanism is due, at least in part, to a direct effect of estrogen on blood vessels is supported in a study performed by Adams et al. [2]. These investigators induced adverse lipoprotein changes in cynomolgus macaque monkeys with an atherogenic diet and high dose estrogen and progestogen oral contraceptives. The coronary arteries in these primates were found to be spared from further atherosclerotic progression despite the adverse lipid changes. This was considered to be secondary to a protective effect of estrogen on the coronary arteries.

Sarrel et al. [3] and others have demonstrated that estrogen improves vascular flow while other studies have confirmed the improvement in arterial pulsatility in the presence of estrogen. The mechanism for this arterial vasodilatation and improved pulsatility index is most likely mediated through prostacyclin synthetase activity. This leads to vasodilatation, improved blood flow, reduced risk of thrombosis and reduced risk of damage due to atherosclerosis.

The action of estrogen in producing vasodilatation and improved blood flow is almost certainly mediated through a classical hormone receptor interaction within cells of the artery wall and within platelets circulating in blood. This hormone-receptor interaction would explain why progestogens occasionally induce a negative or opposing effect on blood flow and dilatation.

Sullivan and colleagues [4] conducted a 10-year retrospective case-control study to determine whether estrogen replacement therapy influenced the prevalence of coronary atherosclerosis as measured by angiographic studies. Two thousand one hundred and eighty-eight postmenopausal women underwent coronary angiography between 1972 and 1984. There were 1444 women who had more than 70% stenosis in one or more of their main coronary arteries and 744 women who had no evidence of any occlusion. The odds ratio estimate of the risk of severe coronary artery disease for estrogen users relative to the risk for nonusers, after adjustment for age, cigarette smoking, diabetes, cholesterol, and hypertension, was 0.44.

Antihypertensive Medications

The aim of antihypertensive drug therapy in postmenopausal women is to reduce the blood pressure to normal levels with the fewest side effects. Ideally, one would choose a therapeutic program which specifically corrects the underlying defect causing the elevated blood pressure. However, as the majority of hypertensive patients will have essential hypertension (> 90% of all cases of hypertension) an empiric approach is used which takes into consideration efficacy, safety, impact on quality of life, and ease of administration.

The guidelines for the treatment of hypertension in most countries recommend five classes of antihypertensive agents as initial therapy, namely beta-blockers, diuretics, alpha-1-receptor blockers, calcium antagonists and angiotensin converting enzyme (ACE) inhibitors. Little evidence exists to show that one is more effective than another, but because of their lower side effects, an increasing number of physicians prefer an ACE inhibitor or a calcium antagonist to be used. For the treatment of essential hypertension in postmenopausal women, ACE inhibitors are emerging as the initial drug of choice. The rationale for this is based on their favourable profile of side effects, where especially postmenopausal women might profit from. However, whether one or another class of antihypertensive agents is more or less favourable for the treatment of hypertension in women has not yet been investigated and has to be proved by controlled studies to be exclusively performed in hypertensive postmenopausal women.

As a gynecologist who is used to treating hypertension in postmenopausal women I would presently choose an ACE inhibitor administered as a once daily dosage as the initial antihypertensive therapy in mild to moderate essential hypertension. ACE inhibitors should be started at a low dose. If arterial pressure is lowered to less than 140/90 mmHg, no further drug therapy is indicated. If the pressure remains elevated, the next step is to increase the dose of the ACE inhibitor. If the blood pressure cannot be controlled by the highest recommended dosis of the ACE inhibitor, then hydrochlorothiazide (HCTZ) should be added. Thiazides potentiate the action of ACE inhibitors. The combination of diuretics with ACE inhibitors is particularly appealing since the adverse metabolic effects of the thiazides, in part, will be ameliorated by the ACE inhibitor. This is not true for beta blockers or calcium antagonists. Indeed beta blockers and thiazides may actually potentiate each others'adverse effects insofar as electrolytes (hypokalemia) and metabolic actions (hypercholesterolemia) are concerned.

If therapy with two drugs does not achieve blood pressure control the primary-care gynecologist is strongly encouraged to refer the patient to a cardiologist or internal medicine specialist.

Conclusions

With increasing life expectancy, many women will spend more than one third of their lifespan in the postmenopausal state. There is now overwhelming evidence that estrogens have an effect not only on improving an atherogenic blood lipid profile, but also on protecting the arterial intima from deposition of cholesterol. From the results of animal studies which have been confirmed by clinical data, most of the protection appears to be mediated at the site of the vessel wall. This protection against atherosclerosis is in the order of 50 %–70 % and results in a reduced risk of death from myocardial infarction, stroke and other cardiac diseases. Angiographic studies also confirm that not only will conjugated equine estrogens help prevent atherosclerosis but, if administered to women who are already severely affected by coronary occlusion, they will also reduce the risk of death from atherosclerotic heart disease.

Although there is evidence that some of the coagulation cascade is tilted in favor of increased coagulation activity, the work of Notelovitz and colleagues [5] is reassuring in that the dosages of natural estrogen administered to postmenopausal women were not associated with an increase in thrombosis.

Many studies confirmed that estrogen not only leads to an increase in blood flow by up to 25 %, but also induces an improvement in the pulsatile index and a consequent fall in blood pressure. For postmenopausal women with chronically elevated blood pressure ACE inhibitors are the first line of therapy.

References

1. Henderson BE, Paganini-Hill A, Ross RK (1991) Decreased mortality in users of estrogen replacement therapy. Arch Intern Med 151:75
2. Adams MR, Clarkson TB, Koritnik DR et al. (1987) Contraceptives, steroids, and coronary artery atherosclerosis in cynomolgus macaques. Fertil Steril 47:1010
3. Sarrel PM, Lindsay D, Rosano GMC, Poole-Wilson PA (1992) Angina and normal coronary arteries in women: gynecologic findings. Am J Obstet Gynecol 167:467
4. Sullivan JM, Vander Zwaag R, Hughes JP et al. (1990) Estrogen replacement and coronary artery disease. Arch Intern Med 150:2557
5. Notelovitz M, Ware M (1982) Coagulation risks with postmenopausal oestrogen therapy. In: Studd J (ed) Progress in obstetrics and gynecology, vol 2. Churchill Livingstone, Edinburgh

Hormone Replacement Therapy and Hypertension: Relationship to the Renin-Angiotensin System

JEAN M. CACCIABAUDO and JEAN E. SEALEY

Introduction

Senaca observed early in the first century A.D., "the illustrious founder of the guild and profession of medicine [Hippocrates] remarked that women never lost their hair or suffered from pain in the feet; and yet nowadays they run short of hair and are afflicted with gout . . . in rivalling male indulgences, they have also rivalled the ills to which men are heirs".

Like Hippocrates, many have assumed that women are less susceptible to male afflictions such as hair loss, gout and heart disease. Seneca made an astute observation: women suffer same ills as men. Cardiovascular disease is the leading cause of death among women in the United States and, in aggregate, more women die from heart disease than men [1]. Nevertheless, this "inheritance" of a man's ills is not related to indulgence but to the natural process of female aging heralded by menopause.

Women in their premenopausal years are rarely afflicted with cardiovascular disease including hypertension. This protection is lost during the postmenopausal years. Since the onset of menopause is marked by the loss of endogenous estrogen production from the ovaries, estrogen is felt to confer the premenopausal protection. Before discussing estrogen replacement therapy and hypertension in postmenopausal women, it is worthwhile to review the hormonal changes that occur during the normal menstrual cycle.

The Menstrual Cycle

Briefly, during the follicular phase of the menstrual cycle, estradiol-17β is secreted by the ovaries in increasing amounts reaching a peak at the time of ovulation (Fig. 1) [2]. Endometrial proliferation occurs in response to stimulation by estradiol-17β. After ovulation, estrogen levels transiently fall but rise again during the luteal phase, in synchrony with the increasing progesterone which is secreted by the corpus luteum. Progesterone stimulates glandular secretion within the endometrial lining. During the premenstrual phase, the corpus luteum regresses and the rates of estradiol-17β and progesterone secretion decrease. Thus, plasma levels of estrogen and progesterone

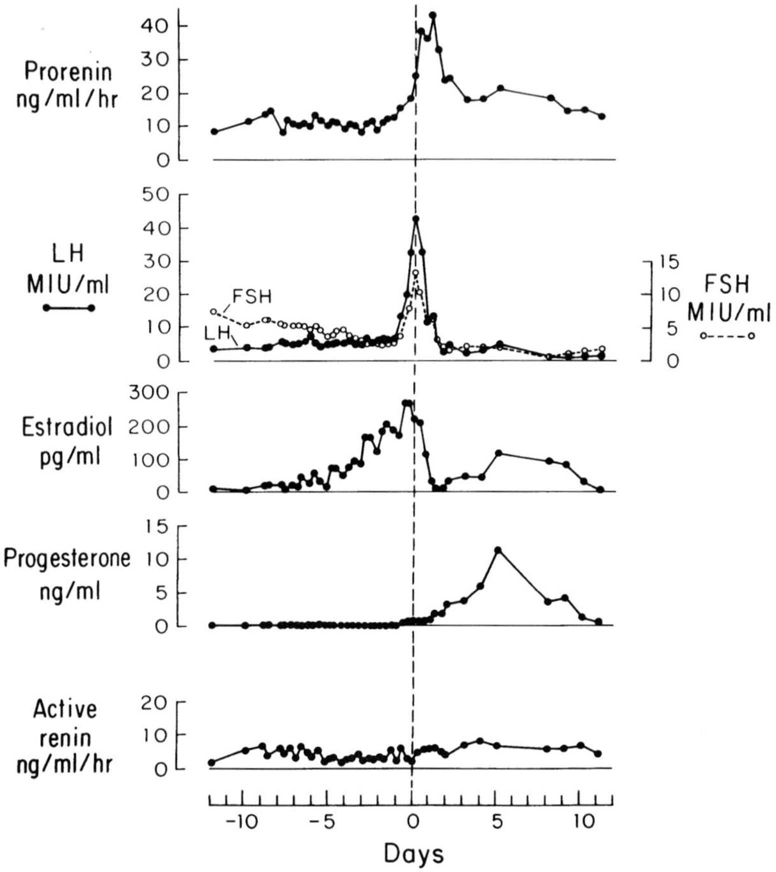

Fig. 1. Hormonal changes during the menstrual cycle. Estradiol peaks at the time of ovulation indicated by day O. *LH*, luteinizing hormone; *FSH*, follicle-stimulating hormone. (From [2])

are never constant. Estrogen levels vary throughout the cycle whereas progesterone rises and falls only during the luteal phase. Plasma renin activity normally does not change during the follicular phase but both renin and aldosterone tend to rise during the luteal phase.

Benefits of Hormone Replacement Therapy

Various regimens of hormone replacement therapy exist. Given the dynamic waxing and waning of sex steroids during the normal menstrual cycle, all these regimens are a poor substitute for the premenopausal state.

Current evidence offers compelling reasons to use hormone replacement therapy for prevention of osteoporosis and protection against cardiovascular disease. Postmenopausal osteoporosis affects 1.5 million people each year. Deficiency of estradiol-17β by natural or surgical menopause results in accelerated bone loss and decreased bone mass. Recent evidence suggests that early estrogen replacement therapy prevents pathologic bone loss by regulating cytokines involved in bone remodeling [3].

Estrogen replacement therapy was not initially given to confer cardioprotection but to protect for osteoporosis and to alleviate unwanted symptoms of menopause such as hot flashes, depression, sleep disturbances, and vaginal dryness. However, epidemiological studies soon began to show beneficial cardiovascular effects. The Nurses' Health Study [4] revealed a 50% decrease in incidence of myocardial infarction in user of estrogens. Both healthy women and those with cardiovascular disease have been shown to benefit from its use. Furthermore, normal replacement doses are beneficial and not additional benefit is gained from using doses higher than 0.625 mg conjugated estrogens or an equivalent dose. This is also the same dose that provides osteoporosis prevention.

Mechanisms Responsible for the Cardioprotective Effects of Female Sex Hormones

There is overwhelming evidence that exogenous estrogens alter lipid metabolism. Nevertheless, it is becoming apparent that this is but one aspect of the impact of estrogens on the cardiovascular system. Estrogen also appears to influence vascular smooth muscle function.

Data suggests that conjugated estrogens increase high-density lipoprotein cholesterol and decrease low-density lipoprotein cholesterol [5]. Estrogens may also have antioxidant effects that protect unsaturated lipids from peroxidation. The antioxidant effects have been attributed to phenolic hydroxyl groups which are found in such estrogens such as estrone, estradiol, and estriol. In vivo studies support the hypothesis that estrogens preserve endothelial integrity and function in the setting of hypercholesterolemia by antioxidant properties [6]. Endothelial function also is influenced by hemostatic factors. Estrogen therapy may decrease plasma fibrinogen and increase plasminogen levels which may contribute to a favorable "cardioprotected" state [7].

It is not readily recognized that estrogen acts as a vasodilator and ultimately may lower blood pressure and increase tissue perfusion. When estradiol is infused locally into uterine circulation of castrated ewes, vascular resistance falls markedly and uterine blood flow increases without change in systemic hemodynamics [8]. Infusion of estradiol-17β systemically into the ewes decreases systemic vascular resistance. Concurrent increases in cardiac output and the renin-angiotensin system result in no net change in mean arteriolar pressure (Fig. 2).

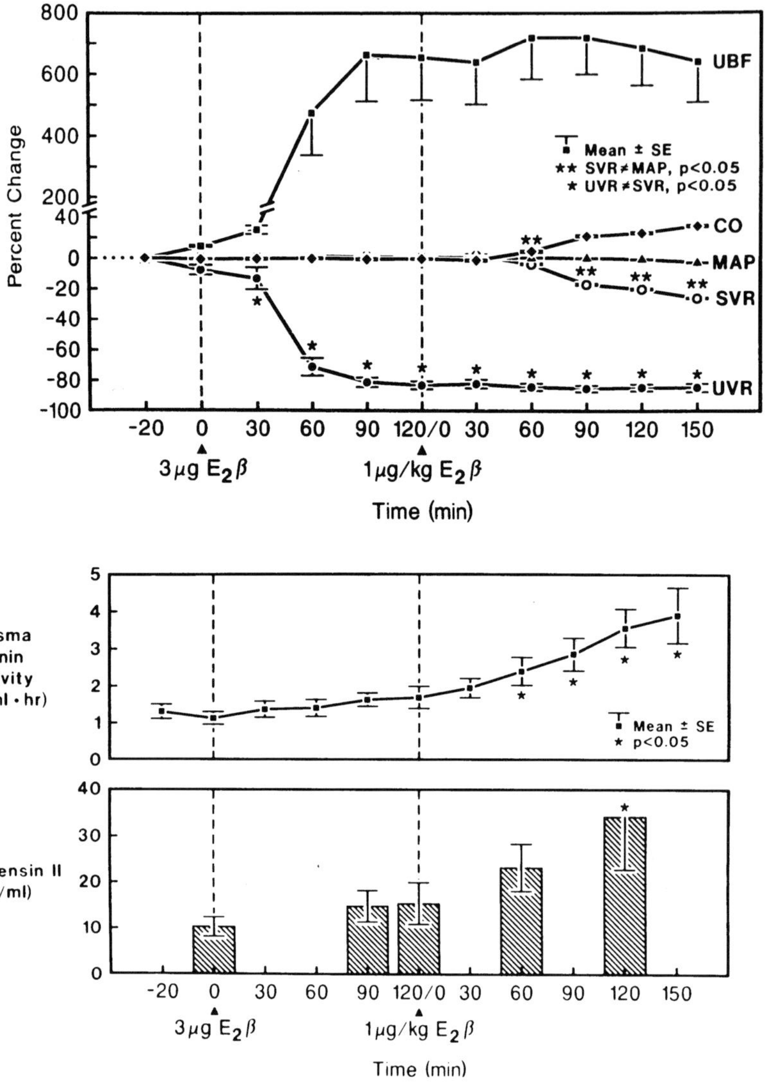

Fig. 2. Effects of local and systemic 17-β estradiol on relative responses of uterine blood flow (*UBF*), cardiac output (*CO*), mean arterial pressure (*MAP*), systemic vascular resistance (*SVR*), uterine vascular resistance (*UVR*), plasma renin activity, and angiotensin II plasma concentration in castrated ewes ($n=5$). (From [8])

Not only does estrogen cause systemic vasodilation but treatment with estradiol-17β may also cause coronary vasodilation. In women performing exercise treadmill tests after administration of sublingual estradiol-17β or placebo there was an increased time to 1 mm ST segment depressions and increased total exercise time [9]. Obviously, myocardial ischemia was improved. This response is reminiscent of the endothelium-dependent effects of nitrates.

Insulin resistance and increased abdominal fat are additional risk factors for cardiovascular disease. Menopause may cause an increase in both. Estrogen treatment is reported to reduce abdominal fat and it may reverse insulin resistance thereby conferring additional cardiovascular protection.

Risk of Hormone Replacement Therapy

Like all medications, there are risks involved in hormone replacement therapy. Unopposed estrogen use causes a six-fold increase in endometrial cancer risk [10]. Addition of progestational agents protect against this risk. The issue of breast cancer risk remains murky with conflicting data. The Nurses' Health Study revealed no increased incidence in breast cancer. On the other hand, a recently published meta-analysis concluded that longterm unopposed estrogen use was associated with a relative risk of 1.25 for developing and dying from breast cancer [11]. Other side effects of hormone replacement therapy include an increased risk of gallbladder disease, as well as bloating, breast tenderness, headache, and depression.

Blood Pressure and Female Sex Hormones

Effects of Oral Contraceptives

The effect of oral contraceptives on blood pressure and cardiovascular disease are in conflict with the beneficial effect of estrogen replacement therapy. In 1967, Laragh et al. [12] reported that 11 hypertensive women on oral contraceptive medication had a lowering in blood pressure after discontinuing use. Since then, combined oral contraceptives have been shown to cause hypertension in 4%–5% of normotensive women and worsen hypertension in 9%–16% with existing hypertension [13, 14]. A review of the data suggests that most women taking oral contraceptives experience a small but detectable increase in both systolic and diastolic blood pressure (Fig. 3) [15, 16].

Effects of Menopause

Aging is associated with an increase in blood pressure. Menopause has been suspected to contribute to this rise and to the development of hypertension in women. A review of the literature on the effects of oral contraceptives and postmenopausal estrogens on systolic blood pressure indicates that the

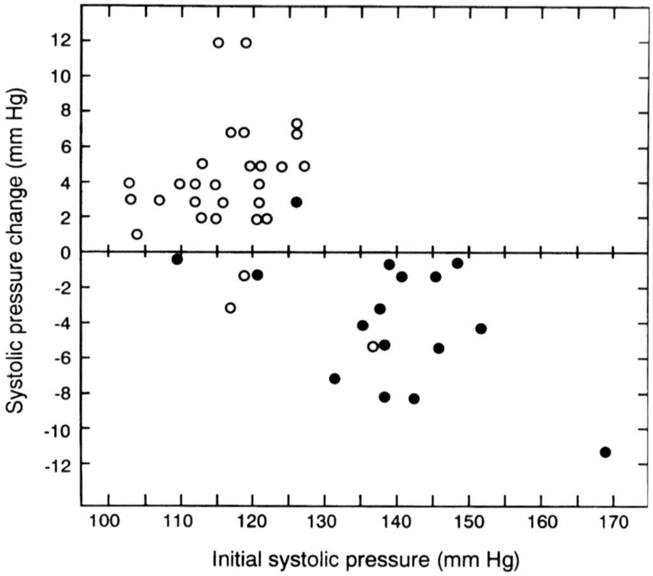

Fig. 3. Effect of oral estrogen in premenopausal women [○] or oral estrogen in postmenopausal women [●] on systolic blood pressure. Summary of longitudinal and cross-sectional studies. (From [16])

postmenopausal women have a higher systolic blood pressure at baseline (Fig. 3) [16]. Nevertheless, longitudinal studies have had difficulties substantiating the sole impact of menopause on blood pressure because of other variables associated with aging including changes in body mass [17].

Effects of Hormone Replacement Therapy

Prospective, randomized clinical trials have shown that in contrast to the effect of oral contraception, normotensive women receiving estrogen therapy tend to have a fall in blood pressure (Fig. 3). Little information is available on the effects of estrogen replacement therapy in hypertensive women, but Luotola [18] describes a lowering of blood pressure in normotensive, hypertensive, and borderline hypertensive women treated with estradiol-17β. However, hemodynamic responses were different in normotensive and hypertensive women. Stroke volume and cardiac output increased in normotensive women. On the other hand, cardiac output fell and peripheral resistance increased in the hypertensive subjects; the reasons for this finding remain unclear.

Like oral contraceptives, there are also reports of blood pressure elevation in some individuals on hormone replacement therapy despite estrogens vasodilatory properties. Analysis of "Pill hypertension" has revealed that plasma renin substrate is increased in all patients taking oral estrogens but the response of plasma renin may be variable [19]. This variability in response of plasma renin activity may offer a clue to the reasons why certain individuals are susceptible to hypertensive effects of estrogen treatment whereas most of the population is not.

Estrogens and the Renin-Angiotensin System

Oral administration of estrogen is associated with elevations of hepatically-metabolized proteins including coagulation factors, lipoproteins, and renin substrate. Intestinal absorption of oral estrogens and entry into the portal circulation result in the liver being exposed to much higher concentrations of estrogen than other organs. This is often referred to as the "first-pass effect".

Percutaneous administration of estrogen is not associated with alterations in hepatically metabolized protein. Thyroid-binding globulin and sex hormone-binding globulin are not elevated by transdermal estrogen nor is renin substrate (angiotensinogen; Fig. 4) [20]. In fact, percutaneous estrogen use in short-term (2 months) studies does not alter lipoprotein levels suggesting that the favorable lipoprotein profile may only result from oral estrogen delivery [21].

Renin substrate (angiotensinogen) is a marker of estrogenic action on the liver. Although renin secretion is the regulated step in the renin system, renin substrate is biochemically rate-limiting since its concentration in plasma allows renin to generate angiotensin I at half maximal velocity. Furthermore, in women on oral contraceptives and elevated renin substrate, plasma renin concentration decreases. Thus, the overall plasma renin activity stays at baseline [22].

In normotensive women on estrogen therapy, blood pressure does not change despite elevations in renin substrate [23]. Under normal physiologic control, the induced increase in angiotensin II production feeds back negatively and reduces the secretion of renin thus maintaining a normal rate of angiotensin II generation and a normal blood pressure. On the other hand, if there is a defect in the feedback control of angiotensin II upon renin secretion, the system resets to a higher rate of angiotensin II production, exerting further vasoconstrictive effects and resulting in an increase in blood pressure. Normally, the rise in blood pressure and sodium retention that accompanies excessive angiotensin II production would also feedback on renin secretion and restore blood pressure to its normal set point. Women with this defective control of renin secretion are at risk for hypertension on estrogen therapy. Thus all women on estrogen therapy require monitoring of blood pressure, especially if hypertension is a preexisting condition. The reciprocal also hold: all hypertensive patients who are taking estrogen replacement therapy should stop estrogen treatment for 2–3 months to determine if blood pressure falls or is more responsive to antihypertensive therapy.

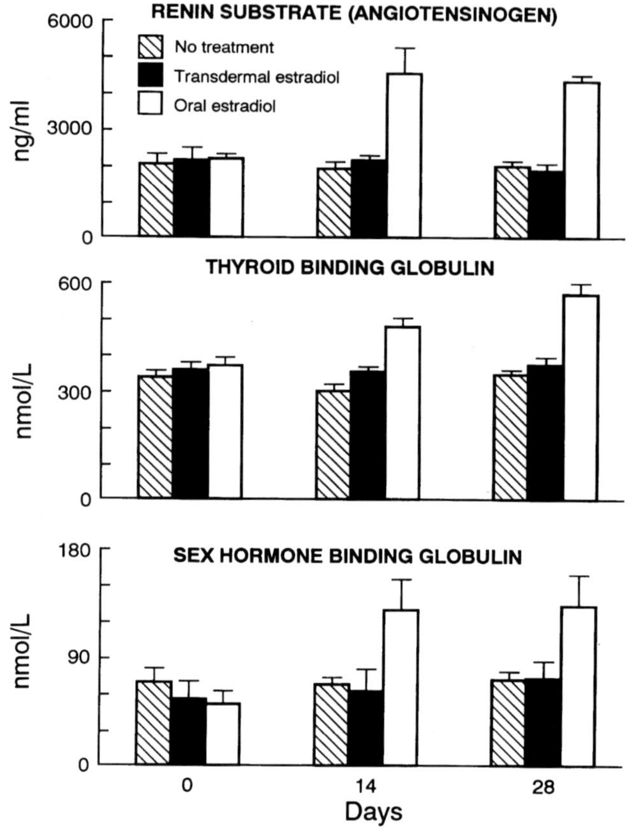

Fig. 4. Comparison of oral and transdermal estradiol administration on renin substrate (angiotensinogen, *top*) and other hepatic proteins (thyroid-binding globulin, *middle*; sex hormone-binding globulin, *bottom*). Oral estradiol raises hepatic protein concentrations indicative of the first-pass effect of oral estrogen. (From [20])

The defect in renin secretion in hypertensive patients is the basis for the hypothesis of nephron heterogeneity in essential hypertensive [24]. In this hypothesis, the hypertensive patient has impaired ischemic nephrons which are intermingled with adapting hyperfiltering hypernatriuretic nephrons. Renin secretion is high from the impaired ischemic nephrons and low from the adapting ones. Inappropriate circulating angiotensin II levels produced by the ischemic nephrons impair sodium excretion from the adapting hyperfiltering nephrons. Plasma renin activity is not inhibited by the eventual elevation in sodium and angiotensin II levels. In such patients, an elevation in angiotensinogen exacerbates the disease.

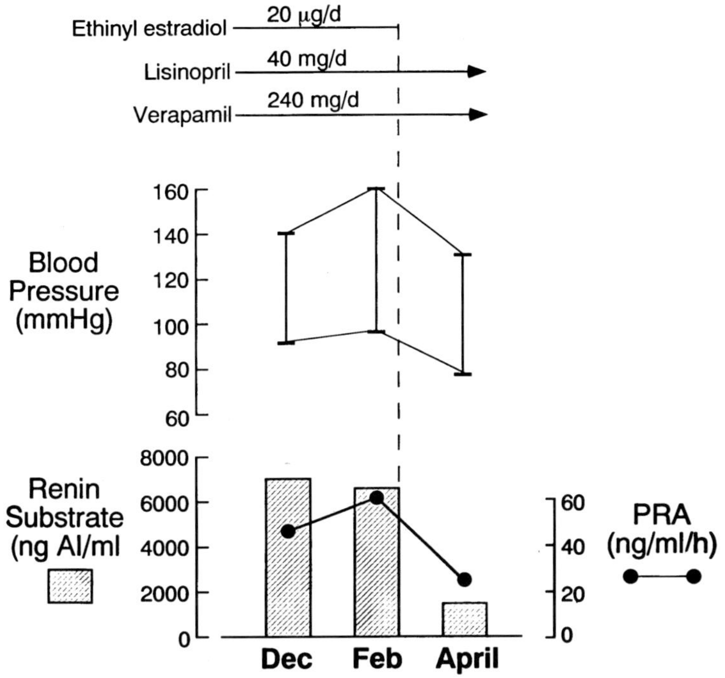

Fig. 5. Effects of hormone replacement therapy cessation on blood pressure in a postmenopausal woman. *PRA*, plasma renin activity

Estrogen, Progesterone and Renin Secretion

Both estrogen and progesterone increase renin secretion. Estrogen via its vasodilator effect and progesterone by competing for the aldosterone receptor resulting in natriuresis [25]. Estrogen also augments the stimulatory effect of progesterone on renin secretion. During the normal menstrual cycle, the estrogen level is not high enough to stimulate renin secretion but progesterone levels do cause a renin rise in many young women during the luteal phase. It is therefore possible that the oral administration of estrogen (and progesterone) may stimulate renin secretion in some women. In those who do not regulate renin secretion normally, this may contribute to the rise in blood pressure.

The early oral contraceptives contained much higher levels of estrogen than currently used. The higher doses may have contributed to the small increase in blood pressure seen in most oral contraceptive users and the occasional development of hypertension in some. Nonetheless, this cannot be the only factor because we occasionally observe a fall in blood pressure in postmenopausal hypertensive patients on hormone replacement therapy upon cessation of hormone replacement therapy (Fig. 5). Estrogen doses are much lower in hormone replacement therapy compared to oral contraceptives.

Summary

Women do not need to be the heirs of man's ills. Therapy with female sex hormones may stave off the threat of cardiovascular disease. The improved lipid profile is, in part, involved in the cardioprotective effects of estrogen treatment, but a fall in blood pressure with increased tissue flow secondary to vasodilatory properties of estrogen confer the majority of benefit. Thus the cardioprotective and anti-osteoporotic effects of hormone replacement therapy in postmenopausal women are valid reasons for its use.

The beneficial effects of estrogen should be weighed against the possibility of endometrial and breast cancer and other adverse effects. Furthermore, blood pressure should be carefully monitored since estrogen and progesterone treatment in susceptible patients can increase blood pressure. The cause appears to be an estrogen-induced 1.5- to fourfold increase in renin-substrate, stimulation of renin secretion by both hormones and subnormal suppression of renin secretion in response to an increased blood pressure. In hypertensive patients taking estrogen replacement therapy, the blood pressure response to withdrawal from hormone replacement therapy should be tested.

As further investigation continues, the unanswered questions of combination estrogen/progesterone effects and percutaneous estrogen effects will be addressed. Nevertheless, current wisdom suggests that, for most patients, postmenopausal hormone replacement therapy is cardioprotective and only the rare patient will develop hypertension.

References

1. Centers for Disease Control and Prevention (1993) Annual summary of births, marriages, divorces, and deaths: United States, 1992. Monthly vital statistics report from the Centers for Disease Control and Prevention, vol 14, pp 1–24
2. Sealey JE, Cholst I, Glorioso N, Troffa C, Weintraub ID, James GD, Laragh JH (1987) Sequential changes in plasma luteinizing hormone and plasma prorenin during the menstrual cycle. J Clin Endocrinol Metab 65:1–5
3. Horowitz MC (1993) Cytokines and estrogen in bone: anti-osteoporotic effects. Science 260:626
4. Colditz GA, Willet WC, Stampfer MJ, Rosher B, Speizer FF, Hennekens CH (1987) Menopause and the risk of coronary heart disease in women. N Engl J Med 316:1105–1110
5. Barrett-Connor E, Bush TL (1991) Estrogen and coronary heart disease in women. JAMA 265:1861–1867
6. Keaney JF, Shwaery GT, Xu A, Nicolosi RJ, Foxall TL, Vita JA (1993) Preservation of endothelial function in hypercholesterolemia through the antioxidant properties of estrogens. Circulation 88:I–79
7. Meilahn EN, Kuller LH, Matthews KAA, Kiss JE (1992) Hemostatic factors according to menopausal status and use of hormone replacement therapy. Ann Epidemiol 2:445–455

8. Magness RR, Rosenfeld CR (1989) Local and systemic estradiol-17beta: effects on uterine and systemic vasodilation. Am J Physiol XX:E536–E542
9. Rosano GMC, Sarrel PM, Poole-Wilson PA, Collins P (1993) Beneficial effect of estrogen on exercise-induced myocardial ischaemia in women with coronary artery disease. Lancet 342:133–136
10. Ravnikar VA (1993) Hormone replacement therapy in the primary prevention of cardiovascular disease: benefits, risks, and compliance issues. In: Wenger NK, Speroff L, Packard B (eds) Cardiovascular health and disease in women. Le Jacq Communications, Greenwich, pp 181–187
11. Grady D, Rubin SM, Petitti DB, Fox CS, Black D, Ettinger B, Ernster VL, Cummings SR (1992) Hormone therapy to prevent disease and prolong life in postmenopausal women. Ann Intern Med 117:1016–1037
12. Laragh JH, Sealey JE, Ledingham JGG, Newton MA (1967) Oral contraceptives: renin, aldosterone and high blood pressure. JAMA 201:918–922
13. Baird DT, Glasier AF (1993) Hormonal contraception. N Engl J Med 328:1543–1549
14. Russel RP, Sullivan MA (1970) The pill and hypertension. Johns Hopkins Med J 127:287–293
15. Woods JW (1988) Oral contraceptives and hypertension. Hyertension 11 [Suppl II]:II.11–II.15
16. McCaffrey TA (1985) Preliminary dissertation. Purdue University, Indiana
17. Van Beresteyn ECH, van 't Hoff MA, de Waard H (1989) Contributions of ovarian failure and aging to blood pressure in normotensive perimenopausal women: a mixed longitudinal study. Am J Epidemiol 129:947–955
18. Luotola H (1983) Blood pressure and hemodynamics in postmenopausal women during estradiol 17-beta substitution. Ann Clin Res 15 [Suppl 38]:1–121
19. Laragh JH (1972) Oral contraceptive hypertension. Postgrad Med 52:98–105
20. Steingold KA, Matt DW, DeZiegler D, Sealey JE, Fratkin M, Reznikov S (1991) Comparison of transdermal to oral estradiol administration on hormonal and hepatic parameters in women with premature ovarian failure. J Clin Endocrinol Metab 73:275–280
21. DeLignieres B, Baevant A (1986) Biological effects of estradiol-17beta in postmenopausal women: oral versus percutaneous administration. J Clin Endocrinol Metab 62:1
22. Derkx FHM, Stuenkel C, Schalekamp MPA, Visser W, Huisveld IH, Schalekamp MADH (1986) Immunoreactive renin, prorenin, and enzymatically active renin in plasma during pregnancy and in women taking oral contraceptives. J Clin Endocrinol Metab 63:1008–1015
23. Hassager C, Riis BJ, Strom V, Guyene TT, Christiansen C (1987) The long-term effect of oral and percutaneous estradiol on plasma renin substrate and blood pressure. Circulation 76:753–758
24. Sealey JE, Blumenfeld JD, Bell GM, Pecker MS, Sommers SC, Laragh JH (1988) On the renal basis for essential hypertension: nephron heterogeneity with discordant renin secretion and sodium excretion causing a hypertensive vasoconstriction-volume relationship. J Hypertension 6:763–777
25. Sealey JE, Itskovitz-Eldor J, Rubattu S, James GD, August P, Thaler I, Levron J, Laragh JH (1993) Estradiol and progesterone related increases in the renin-aldosterone system during ovarian stimulation and early pregnancy (submitted to J Clin Endocrinol Metab)

Is Antihypertensive Therapy Expected to be Different in Postmenopausal Women?

ANNE ZANCHI and HANS R. BRUNNER

Introduction

Coronary heart disease remains the most frequent cause of death among women in the United States and other industrialized countries. Early death after myocardial infarction is higher among women than among men. This may be due to the higher frequency of coexisting diseases or higher age, but delayed care may also be a factor since women undergo fewer invasive procedures for the evaluation of chest pain than men [1, 2].

Postmenopausal women and women who have undergone oophorectomy have a higher risk of coronary heart disease than premenopausal women of similar ages [3]. It is not yet possible to determine exactly why cardiovascular risk is substantially increased in postmenopausal women. The majority of studies revealed a protective effect of hormone replacement therapy on coronary heart disease [4]. This might be related to the favorable effect of the hormone substitution on the lipid profile [5].

The main purpose of this paper is to concentrate on hypertension in postmenopausal women and particularly on their hypertensive treatment.

Hypertension as a Risk Factor in Postmenopausal Women

Systolic blood pressure rises in a nearly linear way with age in men as well as in women. In a longitudinal study from the Framingham cohort, systolic blood pressure was shown to be lower in young women compared to age-matched men but then converged by the age of 60. Diastolic blood pressure in both sexes rises to a peak around 60 years and then decreases. At all ages diastolic blood pressure in women is lower than in men [6].

A prospective trial showed that the change from premenopausal to postmenopausal status does not seem to affect blood pressure, at least not during a follow-up period of 2 1/2 years [7] (Table 1). There was also no significant difference between current hormone users and nonusers in the adjusted mean systolic or diastolic blood pressure [5, 7]. Thus, although hypertension is an important risk factor for cardiovascular disease in postmenopausal women, the age effect on blood pressure does not appear to be noticeably accelerated with the menopause or hormone replacement therapy.

Table 1. Changes in blood pressure (mmHg) in the menopausal and premenopausal women from baseline to follow-up examination (2.5 years)[a]

	Systolic	Diastolic
Baseline		
Menopausal women	110.8 (1.7)	73.1 (0.9)
Premenopausal controls	106.4 (1.3)	71.4 (0.9)
Change at follow-up		
Menopausal women	0.3 (1.2)	1.5 (0.8)
Premenopausal controls	2.4 (1.0)	0.6 (0.7)

[a]From [7]

At all ages, the risk of coronary heart disease remains higher in men than in women for the same levels of blood pressure. This is also the case for stroke; however, the difference between men and women is less pronounced [8] (Table 2).

Women and Pharmacological Trials

Sex-related differences in pharmacokinetics and pharmacodynamics, especially dose response relationships, have been identified for several drugs. These are presumably related to variations in body size, body composition and the effects of sex hormones. In order to ensure that the safety and efficacy of new drugs are well studied in women and in population subgroups defined by such characteristics as age and race, the Food and Drug Administration is changing its policy [9]. Indeed, for instance, the exclusion of women with "childbearing potential" explains the lack of pharmacoki-

Table 2. Average annual incidence (per 1000 subjects) of stroke and transient ischemic attacks by systolic blood pressure (SBP)

SBP (mmHg)	Age (years)			
	35–64		65–94	
	Men	Women	Men	Women
<120	1	1	8	5
120–139	1	1	7	6
140–159	3	2	9	7
160–179	5	2	19	10
> 180	8	5	26	20

netic studies in young women. Many clinical trials have been designed to assess the long-term effect of antihypertensive therapy in men together with pre- and postmenopausal women, who are generally equally represented in the treatment and placebo groups. But almost never are the data analysed in order to detect possible differences in effectiveness or safety between men and women. Prerandomisation stratification according to sex has been recommended by the Food and Drug Administration for large clinical trials in order to distinguish separately the effects of drug therapy according to gender and certainly there will be more data available in the near future. At present however, little information is available on gender related differences in efficacy of antihypertensive drugs.

Trials of Antihypertensive Therapy

Among the clinical trials studying the potential benefits of antihypertensive drug therapy in the elderly the following include men and women.

In the SHEP trial, there is evidence of a favorable effect of active treatment (12.5–25 mg chlortalidone/day with or without 25 mg atenolol/day or 0.05–0.1 mg reserpine/day) on stroke incidence in black and white women over 60 years presenting with isolated systolic hypertension [10]. From the publication, it is however impossible to tell whether the prevention is equally effective in women as in men. Cardiovascular events other than strokes were not even analysed according to gender.

The STOP-H trial, a prospective randomised trial, was conducted to assess the effects of active treatment (β-blockers: atenolol, metoprolol or pindolol; diuretics: hydrochlorothiazide, amiloride) on the frequency of fatal and nonfatal stroke and myocardial infarction in 1627 patients over 60 years with systolic and diastolic hypertension. The active treatment groups experienced a significant 40 % reduction in stroke and a 13 % reduction in myocardial infarction which was not significant. Each sex was equally represented in both groups (63 % of women), but again, data were not analysed or at least not reported according to gender.

A differential analysis with respect to gender was performed recently in the MRC trial [11]. This prospective trial randomised 4396 patients aged 65–74 years to receive diuretic (25–50 mg hydrochlorothiazide/day, 2.5–5 mg amiloride/day), β-blocker (50 mg atenolol) or placebo. Mean follow-up was 5.8 years and the end points were the incidence of strokes, coronary events and deaths from all causes. Over the 5.5 years, 25 % of patients were lost to follow-up, but it is not known whether drug tolerance or side effects were more frequent in women. Overall, the blood pressure response to therapy was the same in men and women. The number of strokes was significantly reduced (25 %) in the active treatment groups (β-blocker and diuretic) and there was no evidence that this effect differed between men and women. There was also a 19 % reduction in coronary artery events and a 17 % reduction in all cardiovascular events which did not differ between both sexes. After adjusting data for baseline characteristics (but not for sex), β-blockade treatment did not induce a significant reduction of these end points. Conversely, the diuretic group was associated with significant reductions in stroke, coronary artery events and all cardiovascular events compared to placebo. Interestingly, the beneficial effects of diuretic therapy were abolished by smoking.

Osteoporosis in Postmenopausal Women

Osteoporosis and its complications associated with fractures is a major public health problem and is one of the important disorders associated with aging [12].

In the United States, it affects more than 20 million individuals, and fractures related to osteoporosis cost the nation an excess of 10 billion U.S. dollars. Hip fracture patients have the highest morbidity of all osteoporosis fracture patients and the mortality at 1 year can reach 30 % [13].

Bone mass is the most accurate predictor of fracture risk. Adult females have less bone mass than men at all ages. The decline of bone mass starts around the fourth decade and is markedly accelerated during the 5 years following menopause [14].

Thus when treating postmenopausal women, every physician should be aware of the risk factors related to osteoporosis in addition to those related to cardiovascular disease. Cigarette smoking, sedentarity and estrogen deficiency states are common risk factors of osteoporosis and cardiovascular disease and the risk reduction with hormone replacement therapy and physical exercise is well documented [15].

Thiazide Treatment

Recently, a lot of attention has been focused on the rate of bone loss and hip fractures in relation with thiazide therapy. Insufficient calcium intake can reduce peak bone mass and enhance aging-associated bone loss. Conversely, long-term thiazide administration reduces the urinary loss of calcium [16].

In a longitudinal study with a mean follow-up of 5 years, the rate of bone loss was significantly reduced among male hypertensive thiazide users (n=325) when compared with normotensive controls (n=639). Antihypertensive therapy other than thiazides had a tendency to increase the rate of bone loss, but this group consisted only of a small number of patients

Table 3. Effects of thiazides and other antihypertensive drugs on rate of bone loss

Treatment	Mean rate of bone loss calcaneus (units/years)	*p* value
Thiazides (*n*=325)	1.50	0.0005
Other drug (*n*=53)	4.22	0.14
Control (*n*=639)	2.95	

(*n*=53) (Table 3) [17]. The beneficial effects of thiazides on the rate of bone loss appears to be dependent on the duration of use. After 2 years treatment with 5 mg bendroflumethiazide/day, the bone mineral content declined at the same rate as in the placebo group although urinary calcium excretion was significantly decreased [18].

The protective effect of thiazides on the incidence of hip fractures was also only apparent after 6 years of treatment. In contrast, antihypertensive diuretic drugs other than thiazide diuretics did not change the relative risk of hip fractures in this retrospective study (905 hip fractures and 5137 population controls) [19].

When the incidence of hip fracture was specifically examined in the postmenopausal female members of the Framingham Study Cohort, pure thiazide users experienced significant protection against hip fracture but not women taking combination drugs containing thiazides. The authors believed that the difference was related to higher doses of thiazides present in the single form of the medication [20]. This fact may also explain the absence in previous studies of any changes in bone mineral density found in all thiazide users [21]. Again, long-term use (> 2 years) strikingly decreased the risk of hip fractures (adjusted odds ratio, 0.27).

When begun soon after menopause, estrogen therapy prevents the early phase of bone loss and decreases the incidence of subsequent osteoporosis-related fractures by about 50% [22]. Additional prospective studies are needed in order to test the real benefit of thiazide therapy on the risk of fracture related osteoporosis, particularly when prescribed in addition to estrogen replacement therapy. Their effects on bone mineral density, the low cost and the proven efficacy in reducing risk of stroke and cardiovascular events should probably favor the use of thiazide diuretics in the treatment of postmenopausal hypertensive women.

Conclusions

Women including postmenopausal women have a lower blood pressure adjusted risk of suffering a major cardiovascular complication than men. However, following a myocardial infarction, the mortality is higher in women than in men. There are very few published data available on the efficacy of antihypertensive drugs in postmenopausal women. It appears that the efficacy of antihypertensive drugs in preventing strokes could be similar in women as in men, but much more data on the prevention of coronary heart disease and stroke in women is needed. Because of the high prevalence of osteoporosis in postmenopausal women and the important morbidity and mortality associated with that disorder, the beneficial effect of thiazide diuretics on the prevention of bone mineral loss and hip fractures seem to favor their use in these patients.

References

1. Steingart RM, Packer M, Hamm P et al. (1991) Sex differences in the management of coronary artery disease. N Engl J Med 325:226–230
2. Wenger NK, Speroff L, Packard B (1993) Cardiovascular health and disease in women. N Engl J Med 329:247–272
3. Kannel WB, Hjortland MC, McNamara PM, Gordon T (1976) Menopause and risk of cardiovascular disease. The Framingham Study. Ann Intern Med 85:447–452
4. Stampfer MJ, Colditz GA (1991) Estrogen replacement therapy and coronary heart disease: a quantitative assessment of the epidemiologic evidence. Prev Med 20:47–63
5. Nabuls AA, Folsom AR, White A, Patsch W, Heiss G, Wu KK, Szklo M (1993) Associatation of hormone-replacement therapy with various cardiovascular risk factors in postmenopausal women. N Engl J Med 328:1069–1075
6. Vokonas PS, Kannel WB, Cupples LA (1988) Epidemiology and risk of hypertension in the elderly: the Framingham Study. J Hypertens 6 [Suppl 1]:S3–S9
7. Mathews KA, Meilahn E, Kuller LH, Kelsey SF, Caggiula AW, Wing RR (1989) Menopause and risk factors for coronary heart disease. N Engl J Med 321:641–646
8. Stokes J, Kannel WB, Wolf PA, D'Agostino RB, Cupples LA (1989) Blood pressure as a risk factor for cardiovascular disease. Hypertension 13 [Suppl I]:I–13–I–18
9. Merkatz RB, Temple R, Sobel S, Feiden K, Kessler DA (1993) Women in clinical trials of new drugs. N Engl J Med 329:292–296
10. Systolic Hypertension in the Elderly Program (SHEP) Cooperative Research Group (1991) Prevention of stroke by antihypertensive treatment in older persons with isolated systolic hypertension: final results of SHEP. JAMA 265:3255–3264
11. Medical Research Council Working Party (1992) Medical Research Council trial of treatment of hypertension in older adults: principal results. Br Med J 304:405–412
12. Riggs BL, Melton JI (1986) Involutional osteoporosis. N Engl J Med 314:1676–1686
13. Sernbo I, Johnell O (1993) Consequences of hip fracture: a prospective study over 1 year. Osteoporosis Int 3:148–153
14. Consensus Development Conference (1993) Diagnosis, prophylaxis, and treatment of osteoporosis. Am J Med 94:646–650
15. Dalsky GP, Stocke KS, Ehsani AA, Slatopolsky E, Lee WC, Birge SJ (1988) Weight-bearing exercise training and lumber bone mineral content in postmenopausal women. Ann Intern Med 108:824–828

16. Middler S, Pak CYC, Murad F, Bartter F (1973) Thiazide diuretics and calcium metabolism. Metabolism 22:139–146
17. Wasnich RJ, Davis J, Ross P, Vogel J (1990) Effect of thiazide on rates of bone mineral loss: a longitudinal study. Br Med J 301:1303–1304
18. Transbol I, Christensen MS, Jensen GF, Christiansen C, MacNair P (1982) Thiazide for the postponement of postmenopausal bone loss. Metabolism 31:383–386
19. Ray WA, Griffin MR, Downey W, Melton LJ (1989) Long-term use of thiazide diuretics and risk of hip fracture. Lancet 1:687–690
20. Felson DT, Sloutskis D, Anderson JJ, Anthony JM, Kiel DP (1991) Thiazide diuretics and the risk of hip fracture. Results from the Framingham Study. JAMA 265:370–373
21. Ooms ME, Lips P, van Lingen A, Valkenburg HA (1993) Determinants of bone mineral density and risk factors for osteoporosis in healthy elderly women. J Bone Miner Res 8:669–675
22. Riggs BL, Melton LJ (1992) The prevention and treatment of osteoporosis. N Engl J Med 27:620–627

Hypertension in Postmenopausal Women: Brief Review of the Literature and Future Research Directions

VERA BITTNER and SUZANNE OPARIL

Introduction

Over 50 million Americans aged 6 and older have hypertension, defined as a blood pressure of 140/90 mmHg or higher [49]. Prevalence is higher in blacks than in whites and hypertension is especially prevalent among the less educated and among lower socioeconomic groups in both races. High blood pressure prevalence increases markedly with age reaching 52.6 % among 55- to 64-year-old American women and 67.5 % among those over age 65 [1]. Prevalence rates of hypertension (BP > 159/94) reported by the WHO MONICA Project among 35- to 64-year-old women in Europe vary widely, as shown in Fig. 1. Hypertension is more common in men than in women in early adulthood and middle age; the reverse is true in the oldest age groups [49] (Fig. 2). Although cross-sectional studies in women find higher blood pressure levels among those who are postmenopausal [46, 56], longitudinal studies have not shown a significant rise in blood pressure at the time of menopause [18, 33, 54]. Improved and more widely applied treatment of hypertension in the United States since the early 1970s has been paralleled by an approximately 40 % decrease in age-adjusted mortality rates from coronary heart disease and a decline of more than 50 % in age-adjusted mortality rates from stroke in black and white women and men [49].

Despite declining mortality trends, cardiovascular disease in women is likely to become an even more important public health problem in the United States in the future. It is estimated that 38 % of women will be 45 years or older by the year 2000, and 45 % of women will be in this age group by the year 2015 [14]. Among 45- to 64-year-old women, one in nine has some form of cardiovascular disease; after the age of 65, this ratio increases to one in three [1]. As the population ages, the number of women dying from cardiovascular disease will thus increase steadily as will health care costs.

Women subjects have been included in a number of trials of antihypertensive therapy, but their numbers have often been too small to allow conclusive subgroup analyses. The available data on hypertension in women has been reviewed in detail elsewhere [6]. This chapter will provide a brief overview of hypertension as a risk factor for cardiovascular disease in women and the impact of antihypertensive therapy and will discuss future research directions.

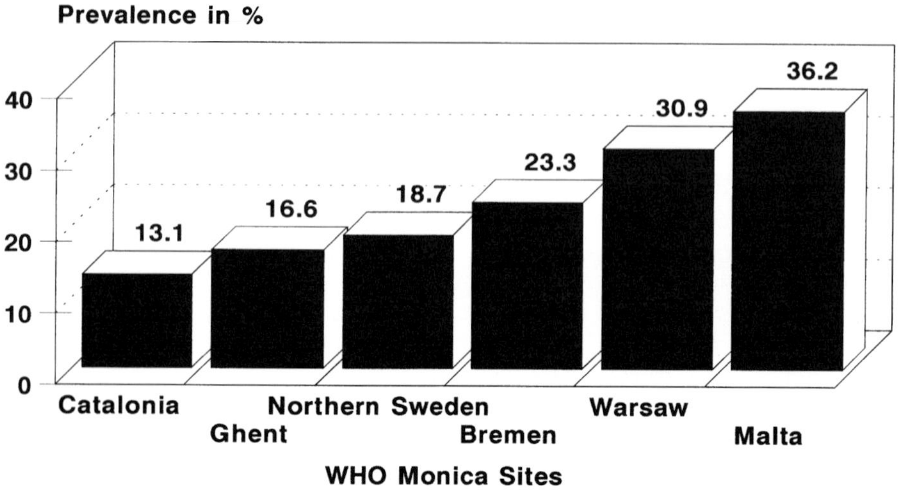

Fig. 1. Prevalence of hypertension in 35- to 64-year-old women reported from selected WHO MONICA sites. Hypertension is defined as blood pressure greater than 159/94 mmHg or antihypertensive treatment. Prevalence ranged from 13.1 % in Catalonia to 36.2 % in Malta [52]

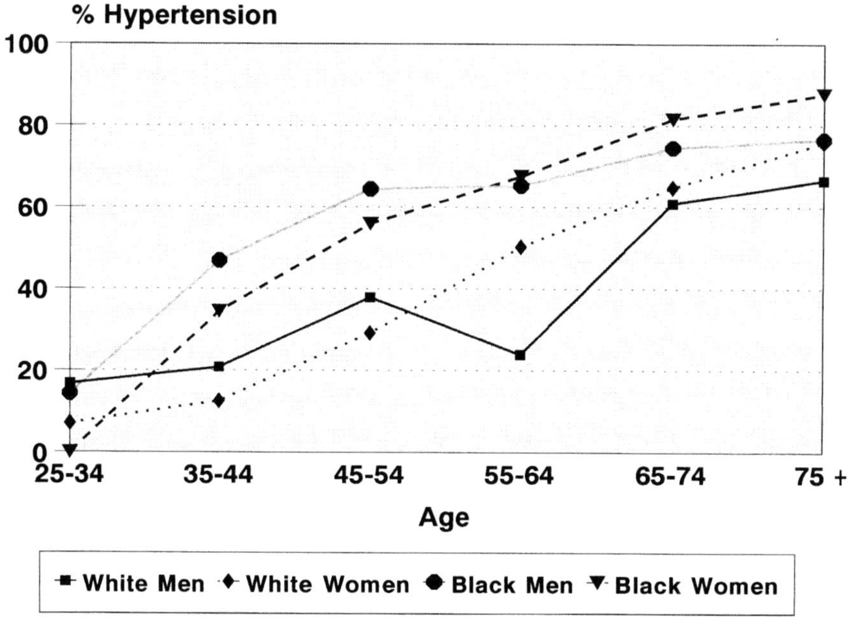

Fig. 2. Prevalence of hypertension by age, race and sex. Prevalence rates rise with age in all race and sex groups. Hypertension is more common in blacks than in whites in most age groups. Under the age of 65, men are more likely to be hypertensive than women, whereas hypertension is more common among women than men in the older age groups [10]

Hypertension as a Risk Factor

Recent data from the NHANES I Epidemiologic Follow-up Study confirm the strong relationship between hypertension and subsequent mortality [10]. The survival analysis included 2616 white men, 2923 white women, 451 black men, and 509 black women. Twelve-year survival rates for persons age 50 and older in all race gender subgroups were lower in individuals with hypertension than in persons with normal blood pressure: 48 % versus 64 % among white men, 68 % versus 82 % among white women, 51 % versus 59 % among black men, and 63 % versus 72 % among black women. This decrease in survival was statistically significant among whites, but not among blacks due to the smaller sample size.

Morbidity due to elevated blood pressure occurs either predominantly as a direct consequence of the elevated intravascular pressure (e.g., in congestive heart failure, aortic dissection, renal insufficiency, and hemorrhagic stroke) or via acceleration of atherosclerosis (coronary heart disease, claudication, atherothrombotic stroke); prognosis worsens when both mechanisms play a role in the patients clinical presentation, e.g., in the patient with marked left ventricular hypertrophy and significant coronary artery disease.

Stroke

Hypertension is strongly related to atherothrombotic and hemorrhagic stroke and is considered the dominant predisposing factor for stroke [13]. The incidence of stroke is about 30 % higher in men than in women and is higher in blacks than in whites.

In the Framingham study, the risk of stroke was proportional to systolic and diastolic blood pressure level in both sexes without a risk threshold [27]. After 30 years of follow-up, systolic hypertension was the most important risk factor for stroke in both sexes [48]. Compared to women with a systolic blood pressure of more than 120 mmHg, 35- to 64-year-old women with a systolic pressure of more than 180 mmHg had a fivefold increase in risk and women between 65 and 94 years of age had a fourfold increase in risk. Left ventricular hypertrophy by ECG was a similarly powerful predictor of stroke: women with left ventricular hypertrophy had a 3.2-fold higher risk of stroke between the ages of 35–64 years and a 5.25-fold higher risk over age 65. Folsom et al. [15] found hypertension to be an independent predictor of stroke among 41837 Iowa women (55–69 years of age), increasing risk of stroke twofold. Pooling data from nine epidemiologic studies (three of which included women subjects), MacMahon et al. [32] estimated that a 7.5 mmHg difference in usual diastolic blood pressure was associated with a 46 % difference in risk of stroke in both sexes.

Cerebral angiography and non-invasive imaging studies have documented a strong link between hypertension and extent of extracranial atherosclerosis. In the Italian Multicenter Study of Reversible Cerebral Ischemic Attacks which included 122 women, systolic blood pressure was the best predictor of extent and severity of extracranial atherosclerosis after adjusting for age and sex; systolic blood pressure did not predict intracranial atherosclerosis [26, 40]. Homer et al. [19] analyzed risk factors among 240 patients (148 men, 92 women) with angiography-proven carotid atherosclerosis: smoking, hypertension, age and LDL-cholesterol were significant predictors of carotid artery atherosclerosis.

The prevalence of carotid atherosclerosis by ultrasound evaluation and its relation to risk factors were assessed in 517 healthy French women between the ages of 45 and 54 years who volunteered for a health check-up [7]. Nearly one third of the women had intimal-medial thickening and 8.7% had atheromatous plaque. Multiple regression analysis revealed that age, smoking, HDL-cholesterol, LDL-cholesterol (or apoprotein B), and systolic (or diastolic) blood pressure were independently related to the severity of carotid atherosclerosis. Hypertension was also a significant risk factor for carotid atherosclerosis in ultrasound studies by Crouse and colleagues [11] and Rubens et al. [43].

Congestive Heart Failure

During 30 years of follow-up of 5070 men and women in Framingham [48], 85 women in the 35- to 64-year-old age group and 144 women in the 65- to 94-year-old age group developed heart failure. In both age groups, women with systolic pressures of more than 180 mmHg were six to seven times more likely to develop heart failure than women with systolic pressures of less than 120 mmHg. An even more striking increase in relative risk of developing heart failure was apparent when women with and without left ventricular hypertrophy were compared (relative risk of 17 in the younger and 6.7 in the older age group, respectively). In this Framingham cohort, 55% of patients with congestive heart failure had a history of hypertension and it was estimated that one third of congestive heart failure could be attributed directly to hypertension [58]. In the current era, hypertension may be less important as an etiologic factor of heart failure. In the Studies of Left Ventricular Dysfunction (SOLVD) Registry, for example, only 7% of patients were classified as having heart failure on the basis of hypertension while over two thirds had heart failure due to ischemic heart disease (unpublished data).

Coronary Heart Disease

Although elevated blood pressure results in altered arterial structure and function and abnormal flow patterns, hypertension alone is not sufficient to induce atherosclerosis [16]. Hypertension in the presence of other risk factors, in particular hypercholesterolemia, clearly accelerates the progression of atherosclerosis [38]. The strong relationship between hypertension and the development of coronary heart disease in Western societies where hypertension and hypercholesterolemia frequently coexist is thus to be expected.

In 14-year follow-up data from the Framingham cohort [28], hypertension was as powerful independent predictor of coronary heart disease in both sexes and the relationship between blood pressure and development of coronary heart disease was graded, without a threshold in risk at lower blood pressure levels. In women, systolic blood pressure was the second (to age) most powerful predictor of coronary heart disease; in men, systolic blood pressure ranked fourth behind age, serum cholesterol, and cigarettes smoked. Systolic blood pressure was also a significant uni- and multivariate predictor of coronary heart disease when follow-up was extended to 30 years [48]. The strength of the relationship varied with age: below age 65, the risk of coronary heart disease at a systolic blood pressure of more than 180 mmHg compared to a systolic blood pressure of 120 mmHg was higher in women (fivefold increase) than in men (threefold increase); in older individuals, the risk was higher in men (fivefold increase) than in women (threefold increase). Left ventricular hypertrophy was an independent contributor to coronary heart disease risk in both sexes, especially among older individuals.

Hypertension was also a strong and independent predictor of myocardial infarction among 18- to 54-year-old women participating in the Walnut Creek Contraceptive Study [41] and among the 40- to 59-year-old women enrolled in the Rochester Coronary Heart Disease Project [5] who were followed for 7 and 23 years, respectively. Assuming a causal relationship between hypertension and coronary heart disease events, the authors in the latter study estimated that hypertension accounted for 45 % of myocardial infarctions and sudden deaths in this cohort.

The relationship between hypertension and coronary heart disease in black women has been the subject of few studies. Tyroler et al. [53] reported coronary heart disease (angina pectoris, myocardial infarction, and sudden death) incidence over 87 months of follow-up for participants in the Evans County Study and did not find a relationship between hypertension and subsequent development of coronary heart disease events in black women. In contrast, investigators in the Charleston Heart Study [29] found low education, systolic pressure and diabetes to be the most predictive variables for fatal and nonfatal coronary heart disease among black women. Furthermore, the risk of dying from coronary heart disease over 25 years of follow-up was increased twofold in these black women with systolic blood pressure of 150 mmHg or more.

Analyzing pooled data from nine epidemiologic studies (including 14611 women and 403732 men), MacMahon et al. [32] found a log-linear relationship between relative risk of coronary heart disease and increasing quintiles of diastolic blood pressure. After adjustment for age, blood cholesterol, and smoking, a 7.5 mmHg difference in usual diastolic blood pressure was associated with a 29% difference in coronary heart disease risk in both sexes.

Although the prevalence of coronary heart disease morbidity and mortality are higher for men than for women over all, the female health advantage is not universal [30]. Women equal or even surpass men in the incidence of certain categories of coronary disease, such as angina pectoris, and the prognosis of women with established coronary heart disease is worse than that of men. Women of all ages are at higher risk of death during an acute myocardial infarction than are age matched men. The male-female differential in coronary heart disease morbidity and mortality has been attributed to gender differences in cardiovascular risk factors. For example, cigarette smoking is more prevalent among men, while high-density lipoprotein (HDL) cholesterol levels are higher among women. In addition, there are gender differences in the impact of some of the risk factors on cardiovascular morbidity and mortality. The most dramatic example of this is diabetes mellitus: diabetic women are at three fold greater risk of cardiovascular death than diabetic men [30]. This difference persists even when adjusted for other risk factors, including age, blood pressure, cholesterol levels, cigarette smoking and left ventricular hypertrophy by electrocardiogram. Thus, the presence of diabetes abolishes and even reverses the gender differential in cardiovascular risk. The occurrence of the menopause, whether natural or surgically induced, is also associated with an escalation in cardiovascular risk. This appears to be due to a combination of worsening of circulating lipoprotein levels, principally decreases in HDL, and adverse effects of estrogen withdrawal on endothelial cell biology. Further investigation is needed to define the mechanisms by which the menopause enhances cardiovascular risk and to determine whether postmenopausal estrogen replacement can protect the cardiovascular system from these alterations.

Impact of Antihypertensive Therapy

Clinical Trials

In more than 95% of cases of human hypertension, the cause(s) of elevated blood pressure cannot be identified. Epidemiologic and genetic segregation studies strongly suggest that hypertension is inherited as a polygenic disease, but the genes involved have not yet been identified. Factors that have been implicated in the genesis of essential hypertension include increased sympathetic nervous system activity, increased or "inappropriate" renin secretion, overproduction of an unidentified Na^+-retaining hormone, chronic high Na^+ intake, inadequate dietary intakes of K^+ and Ca^{2+}, deficiencies of vasodilators such as prostacyclin, atrial natriuretic peptide and endothelium derived relaxing factor (nitric oxide), excesses of vasoconstrictors such as angiotensin II, endothelin and thromboxane, congential abnormalities of the resistance vessels, diabetes mellitus, insulin resistance, obesity, increased activity of vascular growth factors, and altered cell ion transport [39].

These different pathophysiologic mechanisms have not been taken into account in the design of large scale trials of antihypertensive therapy performed over the last 30 years [2, 3, 9, 12, 17, 20–25, 34–36, 42, 44, 45, 50, 51, 55]. Non-hemodynamic effects of antihypertensive agents have also not been considered; rather, choice of agents was determined by considerations of safety and efficacy in lowering of blood pressure and doses of antihypertensives were titrated according to hemodynamic response. The trials differ significantly in the type and intensity of pharmacologic therapy, inclusion and exclusion criteria, and study endpoints; only 3 trials did not include women [17, 36, 55]. In addition to reporting overall morbidity and mortality statistics, some studies have attempted to analyze data in women separately [3, 9, 20–21, 23–25, 35, 44–45], but none of these trials included enough women to convincingly analyze gender subgroups. Not surprisingly, these subgroup analyses have yielded variable results regarding the risk/benefit ratio of pharmacological treatment of hypertension in women, particularly in white women.

The Hypertension Detection and Follow-up Program (HDFP). This trial [20–25, 44] had a unique design in that it compared community based management of diastolic hypertension (referred care, RC) with a more intensive, fixed-protocol, study clinic based approach (stepped care, SC). The SC protocol used chlorthalidone alone or in combination with reserpine, hydralazine, guanethidine, or other antihypertensive agents if needed. There was no placebo group. Out of 10940 subjects age 30–69 years, 1344 black and 1185 white women were assigned to the SC arm, and 1354 black and 1156 white women to the RC arm. After 5 years, mortality among black women in the SC group was 27.8 % lower than in black women in the RC group, while white women in the SC group had a paradoxical 2.1 % increase in mortality. When follow-up was extended to 6.7 years [38], the apparent adverse effect of SC on white women was no longer present. White SC women had a 22 % lower mortality than white women in the RC group, while black SC women had a 15 % reduction. The survival advantage persisted in all race and sex groups to the 8.3 year follow-up point, with higher relative reductions in mortality in blacks than in whites.

Total stroke rates in HDFP were lower in all race/gender subgroups in the SC arm at 5 years. After adjusting for age and entry diastolic blood pressure, white women in the SC group experienced a 30.4 % reduction in fatal and non-fatal strokes and black women had a 45.5 % reduction. The relative reduction in stroke rates was highest (50 %) in those without prior endorgan damage and without pre-trial antihypertensive therapy. The 5-year incidence of fatal coronary heart disease and nonfatal myocardial infarction was 15.2 % lower among women in the SC group compared to women in the RC group.

The Australian Therapeutic Trial in Mild Hypertension. This trial [42] was a randomized, placebo controlled study involving 3427 white individuals (1257 women) 30–69 years old with a diastolic blood pressure of more than 95 mmHg but less than 110 mmHg and systolic blood pressure of more than 200 mmHg who did not have any preexisting cardiovascular disease. Pharmacological therapy in the active treatment group consisted of chlorothiazide and, if necessary, a second-line (propranolol, alpha-methyl-dopa, pindolol) and a third-line agent (hydralazine, clonidine) to achieve an initial diastolic blood pressure of less than 90 mmHg and to further decrease the diastolic pressure to less than 80 mmHg at the 2-year point. Both fatal (all cause mortality, cardiovascular mortality) and non-fatal end points (stroke, transient ischemic attack, myocardial infarction, other ischemic heart disease, heart failure, aortic dissection, retinopathy, encephalopathy, renal insufficiency) were analyzed after 4 years of follow-up. By intention to treat analysis, there were significant reductions in cardiovascular deaths and in the combined category "all trial endpoints" in the active treatment group (57.7 % and 19.6 %, respectively). Cerebrovascular events were reduced significantly (17 versus 31 events, $p < 0.025$), but there was no difference in ischemic heart disease events (98 versus 109 events in active and placebo groups, respectively). A significant reduction in cumulative all cause mortality in the active treatment group was apparent when only patients adhering to the trial regimen were analyzed. Upon initial analysis, treatment benefit appeared to be restricted to men, but Cox proportionate hazards analysis in a subsequent paper confirmed a significant treatment benefit in women, esp. among older women smokers [50].

The Study by the European Working Party (EWP). This trial [2, 3] included 840 subjects (70 % women) with a mean age of 72 years who had diastolic blood pressures of 90–119 mmHg and systolic pressures of 160–239 mmHg in a double-blind randomized design comparing hydrochlorothiazide/triamterene (if necessary supplemented with alpha-methyl-dopa) and placebo with a mean follow-up of 4.7 years. Mortality analysis was by intention to treat. All cause mortality was not changed by therapy, but cardiovascular mortality decreased by 27 % (p=0.037) due to a significant decrease in cardiac mortality (-38 %, p=0.036) and a statistically nonsignificant decrease in cerebrovascular mortality (-32 %).

When events were analyzed by gender, women had an 18 % (not statistically significant) reduction in cardiovascular mortality while men had a statistically significant 46 % reduction. Both men and women had a significant 44 % reduction in cardiovascular study terminating events. Multivariate Cox proportional hazards analysis suggested that the effect of therapy was not gender dependent, but that there was an age dependence in that individuals over 80 years of age did not seem to benefit from treatment. Since 90 % of the 155 individuals over age 80 were women, this may partially explain the lesser treatment effect on cardiovascular mortality in women.

The Medical Research Council (MRC) Trial. This trial [35] was a single-blind, general practice based British trial involving 17 354 patients (8306 women) aged 35–64 years with diastolic blood pressure between 90 and 105 mmHg and systolic blood pressures of less than 200 mmHg. Patients with recent cardiovascular events, heart failure, angina and diabetes mellitus were excluded. Patients were randomized to receive either active treatment (bendrofluazide or propanolol with or without additional alpha-methyl-dopa) or placebo and were followed for 5.5 years. Diastolic blood pressure was approximately 5 mmHg lower in the active treatment group than in the placebo group; only 70 % of individuals in the active treatment group achieved the diastolic blood pressure goal of 90 mmHg or less, while 40 % achieved this level in the placebo group. There were no statistically significant differences in all cause mortality or coronary events between groups, although the trends favoured the active treatment group. There were significant reductions in stroke rate (-46 %) and incidence of all cardiovascular events (-18 %) in the active treatment group compared to the placebo group. In a posthoc gender subgroup analysis, all cause mortality was significantly reduced among men in the active treatment group (7.1 versus 8.2 deaths per 1000 person years), while women in the active treatment group had a higher mortality rate than in the placebo group (4.4 versus 3.5 deaths per 1000 person years). There were no gender differences in the other trial endpoints.

The Systolic Hypertension in the Elderly Program (SHEP). This trial [45, 51] was a randomized double-blind placebo controlled trial in 4736 elderly (> 60 year old) individuals (2690 women; 440 black, 2250 white) with a 4.5-years follow-up period which assessed the effects of treatment of isolated systolic hypertension (diastolic blood pressure < 90 mmHg; systolic blood pressure 160–219 mmHg) using chlorthalidone with or without low dose atenolol. The prevalence of cardiovascular and cerebrovascular disease at entry was low. Treatment goals as specified in the protocol were achieved in 70 % of patients in the active treatment group and in 44 % of those in the placebo group (by year 5, 44 % of placebo patients were on antihypertensive therapy). The primary endpoint of the study was the combined incidence of fatal and nonfatal stroke; multiple secondary endpoints relating to cardiovascular morbidity and mortality, and quality of life measures were also assessed. Overall stroke rate was reduced by 36 % with lower incidence rates in all age groups and all blood pressure levels. Gender analysis showed favorable effects in both black (seven versus 21 events) and white women (48 versus 64 events). Analysis of secondary cardiovascular endpoints revealed significant reductions in fatal plus nonfatal coronary heart disease events (RR, 0.73; 95 % Cl, 0.57, 0.94) and fatal plus nonfatal cardiovascular events (RR, 0.68; 95 % Cl, 0.58, 0.79) as well as favorable trends in all cause mortality, total cardiovascular deaths and total coronary heart disease deaths. Gender-specific data for these secondary endpoints are not available.

The Swedish Trial in Old Patients with Hypertension (STOP-Hypertension). This trial [12] was a prospective, randomized, double-blind trial of antihypertensive therapy in 1,627 elderly patients (63 % women) who were between 70 and 84 years old at entry and had either systolic pressures of more than 180 mmHg with diastolic pressures of 90 mmHg or more or diastolic pressures of more than 105 mmHg irrespective of systolic blood pressure. Individuals with isolated systolic hypertension, severe systolic (> 230 mmHg) or diastolic hypertension (> 120 mmHg), orthostatic hypotension, and recent (within the last 12 months) myocardial infarction or stroke were excluded. Treatment consisted of either atenolol (50 mg), hydrochlorothiazide plus amiloride (25/2.5 mg), metoprolol (100 mg), pindolol (5 mg), or a combination of diuretic and beta-blocker. Two thirds of actively treated patients received combination therapy. The study was terminated by the Safety Committee after a mean follow-up time of 25 months because of a significantly lower incidence of fatal and nonfatal stroke, fatal and nonfatal myocardial infarction, and other cardiovascular death (the primary study endpoint) among actively treated individuals compared to placebo treated patients (relative risk, 0.6; 95 % CI, 0.43, 0.85). Further, the incidence of fatal plus nonfatal stroke and all cause mortality were also significantly lower in patients on antihypertensive therapy (relative risk for the latter, 0.57; 95 % CI, 0.37, 0.87) and secondary endpoints such as congestive heart failure, uncontrolled hypertension, transient ischemic attacks, and angina pectoris were less frequent in actively treated patients (40 events versus 132 events, $p<0.001$). The benefical effects of antihypertensive therapy were evident at all ages studied. A gender-specific analysis was not performed.

Pooled Results. MacMahon and colleagues [31] pooled the gender-specific results of the HDFP and MRC trials. The likelihood of detecting statistically significant treatment effects in women was found to be reduced because of lower event rates among women in the control groups of both trials. Nevertheless, the observed 4 % decrease in overall mortality in treated women (95 % CI, -20 % to +16 %) was not significantly different from that seen in men (17 % reduction; 95 % CI, -27 % to -4 %) and the incidence of fatal and nonfatal stroke was significantly reduced in treated women (43 % reduction; 95 % CI, –57 % to –23 %), a benefit similar to that seen in treated men (37 % reduction; 95 % CI, –51 % to –19 %). Coronary event rates were not pooled because of different endpoint definitions in the two studies.

Role of Postmenopausal Hormone Replacement Therapy

In contrast to the experience with oral contraceptives, adverse effects on blood pressure with postmenopausal hormone replacement are rare [49]. The data from Rancho Bernardo suggest that combination therapy with an estrogen and progestin may even result in slight lowering of blood pressure; a similar effect was not seen with estrogen therapy alone [4]. The more recent report from the Atherosclerosis Risk in Communities Study (ARIC) did not find any differences in blood pressure between hormone users and nonusers [37]. Blood pressure lowering is thus not a likely mechanism for the approximately 50 % reduction in coronary heart disease events seen in observational studies of hormone replacement therapy [8, 47]. This protective effect is believed to be due predominantly to favorable effects on serum lipoprotein patterns [8], but direct effects of hormones and in particular estrogen on vascular endothelium and smooth muscle cells may play a significant role [57]. Interactions between hormone replacement therapy and antihypertensive agents have not been explored.

Future Research Directions

Studies to date have emphasized correction of the hemodynamic abnormalities in patients with hypertension and have been successful in preventing the sequelae of these hemodynamic abnormalities including renal disease, congestive heart failure, and stroke. The reduction in coronary heart disease events for any given reduction in blood pressure has been less than that predicted from observational studies, possibly related to adverse effects of antihypertensive agents on the metabolic abnormalities which so often coexist in patients with hypertension including insulin resistance, glucose intolerance, and dyslipidemia. The Antihypertensive and Lipid Lowering to Prevent Heart Attack Trial (ALLHAT) which is currently in the planning stage has been specifically designed to test the hypothesis that newer antihypertensive agents such as calcium channel blockers, ACE-inhibitors, and alphablockers will be more effective in lowering the incidence of coronary heart disease than thiazide-type diuretics. Enrollment of 22 000 men and 18 000 women age 60 and older with 55 % African-American representation is anticipated. Although power calculations suggest that definitive subgroup analyses will not be possible, differential effects of these antihypertensive agents in women and men and blacks and whites may become apparent.

Recruitment for the Women's Health Initiative (WHI) has recently begun. The hormone replacement therapy branch of WHI is designed to assess the effect of hormone replacement therapy on subsequent development of cardiovascular disease in postmenopausal women. Women with severe hypertension (systolic blood pressure $<$ 200 mmHg; diastolic blood pressure < 105 mmHg) are specifically excluded from the trial. It will be possible, however, to gather data on the effects of hormone replacement therapy on blood pressure in normotensive and mildly to moderately hypertensive women and to determine the effect on other risk factors for coronary heart disease in these subgroups. Substudies could be designed to explore the interaction of antihypertensive therapy and hormone replacement therapy. The dietary modification branch of WHI is designed to assess the effects of a "20% fat/high fruit and fiber diet" on breast cancer, colorectal cancer, and coronary heart disease. Weight loss, improvement in lipoprotein profiles, and reduction in blood pressure levels are anticipated and should lead to a lowering of coronary heart disease incidence. It will be possible to compare the efficacy of diet modification in lowering blood pressure levels and cardiovascular risk in white and black participants and different age groups, to assess the effect of diet on dosage requirements of antihypertensive agents, and to explore possible synergism between pharmacologic therapy of hypertension and dietary fat restriction.

As in men, there is marked heterogeneity in pathophysiologic mechanisms of hypertension among women. Cost-effective and practical clinical tests must be developed to classify patients according to the underlying pathophysiologic abnormality(ies) so that therapy can be tailored to each individual patient. This more specific therapy is likely to have a greater impact on coronary heart disease risk than the currently recommended universal step-care approach to hypertension.

References

1. American Heart Association (1993) Heart and stroke facts statistics. American Heart Association
2. Amery A, Birkenheager W, Brixxo P, Bulpitt C, Clement D, Deruyttere M, De Schaepdryver A, Dollery C, Fagard R, Forette F, Forte J, Hamdy R, Henry JF, Joossens JV, Leonetti G, Lund-Johansen P, O'Malley K, Petrie K, Strasser T, Tuomilehto J, Williams B (1985) Mortality and morbidity results from the European Working Party on High Blood Pressure in the Elderly Trial. Lancet 1:1349–1354
3. Amery A, Birkenhaeger W, Brixxo P, Bulpitt C, Clement D, Deruyttere M, De Schaepdryver A, Dollery C, Fagard R, Forette F, Forte J, Hamdy R, Henry JF, Joossens JV, Leonetti G, Lund-Johansen P, O'Malley K, Petrie K, Strasser T, Tuomilehto J, Williams B (1986) Efficacy of antihypertensive drug treatment according to age, sex, blood pressure, and previous cardiovascular disease in patients over the age of 60. Lancet 2:589–592
4. Barrett-Connor E, Wingard DL, Criqui MH (1989) Postmenopausal estrogen use and heart disease risk factors in the 1980s. Rancho Bernardo, Calif, Revisited. JAMA 261:2095–2100
5. Beard CM, Kottke TE, Annegers JF, Ballard DJ (1989) The Rochester Coronary Heart Disease Project: effect of cigarette smoking, hypertension, diabetes, and steroidal estrogen use on coronary heart disease among 40-to 59-year-old women, 1960 through 1982. Mayo Clin Proc 64:1471–1480

6. Bittner V, Oparil S (1993) Hypertension. In: Douglas PS (ed) Cardiovascular health and disease in women. Saunders, Philadelphia, pp 63–104
7. Bonithon-Kopp C, Scarabin PY, Taquet A, Touboul PJ, Malmejac A, Guize L (1991) Risk factors for early carotid artherosclerosis in middle-aged French women. Arteriosclerosis Thrombosis 11:966–972
8. Bush TL, Barrett-Connor E, Cowan LD, Criqui MH, Wallace RB, Suchindran CM, Tyroler HA, Rifkind BM (1987) Cardiovascular mortality and noncontraceptive use of estrogen in women: results from the Lipid Research Clinics Program Follow-up Study. Circulation 75:1102–1109
9. Coope J, Warrender TS (1986) Randomised trial of treatment of hypertension in elderly patients in primary care. Br Med J 293:1145–1151
10. Cornoni-Huntley J, LaCroix AZ, Havlik RJ (1989) Race and sex differentials in the impact of hypertension in the United States. The National Health and Nutrition Examination Survey I Epidemiologic Follow-up Study. Arch Intern Med 149:780–788
11. Crouse JR, Toole JF, McKinney WM, Dignan MB, Howard G, Kahl FR, McMahan MR, Harpold GH (1987) Risk factors for extracranial carotid artery atherosclerosis. Stroke 18:990–996
12. Dahloef B, Lindholm L, Hansson L, Schersten B, Ekbom T, Wester P-O (1991) Morbidity and mortality in the Swedish Trial in Old Patients with Hypertension (STOP-Hypertension). Lancet 338:1281–1285
13. Dyken ML, Wolf PA, Barnett HJM, Bergan JJ, Hass WK, Kannel WB, Kuller L, Kurtzke JF, Sundt TM (1984) Risk factors in stroke. A statement for physicians by the Subcommittee on Risk Factors and Stroke of the Stroke Council. Stroke 15:1105–1111
14. Eaker ED, Chesebro JH, Sacks FM, Wenger NK, Whisnant JP, Winston M (1993) Cardiovascular disease in women. Circulation 88:1999–2009
15. Folsom AR, Prineas RJ, Kaye SA, Munger RG (1990) Incidence of hypertension and stroke in relation to body fat distribution and other risk factors in older women. Stroke 21:701–706
16. Heistad DD, Lopez JAG, Baumbach GL (1991) Hemodynamic determinants of vascular changes in hypertension and atherosclerosis. Hypertension 17[Suppl III]:III75–III11
17. Helgeland A (1982) Treatment of mild hypertension: a five year controlled drug trial. The Oslo Study. Am J Med 69:725–732
18. Hjörtland MC, McNamara PM, Kannel WB (1976) Some atherogenic concommitants of menopause: the Framingham Study. Am J Epidemiol 103:304–311
19. Homer D, Ingall TJ, Baker HL, O'Fallon WM, Kottke BA, Whisnant JP (1991) Serum lipids and lipoproteins are less powerful predictors of extracranial carotid artery atherosclerosis than are cigarette smoking and hypertension. Mayo Clin Proc 66:259–267
20. Hypertension Detection and Follow-up Program Cooperative Group (1979) Five-year findings of the Hypertension Detection and Follow-up Program. Mortality by race, sex, and age. JAMA 242:2572–2577
21. Hypertension Detection and Follow-up Program Cooperative Group (1982) Five-year findings of the Hypertension Detection and Follow-up Program. Reduction in stroke incidence among persons with high blood pressure. JAMA 247:633–638
22. Hypertension Detection and Follow-up Program Cooperative Group (1982) The effect of treatment on mortality in mild hypertension. N Engl J Med 307:976–980
23. Hypertension Detection and Follow-up Program Cooperative Group (1984) Effect of stepped care treatment on the incidence of myocardial infarction and angina pectoris. 5-year findings of the Hypertension Detection and Follow-up Program. Hypertension 6[Suppl 1]:198–206
24. Hypertension Detection and Follow-up Program Cooperative Group (1985) Five-year findings of the Hypertension Detection and Follow-up Program. Pre-

vention and reversal of left ventricular hypertrophy with antihypertensive therapy. Hypertension 7:105–112
25. Hypertension Detection and Follow-up Program Cooperative Group (1988) Persistence of reduction in blood pressure and mortality of participants in the Hypertension Detection and Follow-up Program. JAMA 259:2113–2122
26. Inzitari D, Bianchi F, Pracucci G, Albanese V, Argentino C, Bono G, Brambilla GL, Candelise L, De Zanche L, Mariani F, Passero S, Prencipe M, Fieschi C (1986) The Italian Multicenter Study of Reversible Cerebral Ischemic Attacks. IV. Blood pressure components and atherosclerotic lesions. Stroke 17:185–191
27. Kannel WB, Wolf PA, Verter J, McNamara PM (1970) Epidemiologic assessment of the role of blood pressure in stroke. The Framingham Study. JAMA 214:301–310
28. Kannel WB, Gordon T, Schwartz MJ (1971) Systolic versus diastolic blood pressure and risk of coronary heart disease. The Framingham Study. Am J Cardiol 27:335–346
29. Keil JE, Tyroler HA, Gazes PC (1991) Predictors of coronary heart disease in blacks. Cardiovasc Clin 21:227–239
30. Lerner DJ, Kannel WB (1986) Patterns of coronary heart disease morbidity and mortality in the sexes: a 26-year follow-up of the Framingham population. Am Heart J 111:383–390
31. MacMahon SW, Cutler JA, Furberg CD, Payne GH (1986) The effects of drug treatment for hypertension on morbidity and mortality from cardiovascular disease: a review of randomized controlled trials. Prog Cardiovasc Dis 29[Suppl 1]:99–118
32. MacMahon S, Peto R, Cutler J, Collins R, Sorlie P, Neaton J, Abbott R, Godwin J, Dyer A, Stamler J (1990) Blood pressure, stroke and coronary heart disease. 1. Prolonged differences in blood pressure: prospective observational studies corrected for the regression dilution bias. Lancet 335:765–774
33. Matthews KA, Meilahn E, Kuller LH, Kelsey SF, Caggiula AW, Wing RR (1989) Menopause and risk factors for coronary heart disease. N Engl J Med 321:641–646
34. McFate Smith W (1977) Treatment of mild hypertension. Results of a ten-year intervention trial. U.S. Public Health Service Hospitals Cooperative Study Group. Circ Res 40[Suppl I]:98–105
35. Medical Research Council Working Party (1985) MRC trial of treatment of mild hypertension. Principal results. Br Med J 291:97–104
36. Multiple risk factor intervention trial (1982) Risk factor changes and mortality results. JAMA 248:1465–1477
37. Nabulsi AA, Folsom AR, White A, Patsch W, Heiss G, Wu KK, Szklo M, for the Atherosclerosis Risk in Communities Study Investigators (1993) Association of hormone-replacement therapy with various cardiovascular risk factors in postmenopausal women. N Engl J Med 328:1069–1075
38. O'Kelly BF, Massie BM, Tubau JF, Szlachcic J (1989) Coronary morbidity and mortality, pre-existing silent coronary artery disease, and mild hypertension. Ann Intern Med 110:1017–1026
39. Oparil S (1992) Arterial hypertension. In: Wyngaarden JB, Smith LH Jr, Bennett JC (eds) Cecil's textbook of medicine. Saunders, Philadelphia, pp 253–269
40. Passero S, Rossi G, Nardini M, Bonelli G, D'Etorre M, Martini A, Battistini N, Albanese V, Bono G, Brambilla GL, Candelise L, De Zanche L, Inzitari D, Rasura M, Fieschi G (1987) Italian Multicenter Study of Reversible Cerebral Ischemic Attacks. 5. Risk factors and cerebral atherosclerosis. Atherosclerosis 63:211–224
41. Petitti DB, Wingerd J, Pellegrin F, Ramcharan S (1979) Risk of vascular disease in women. Smoking, oral contraceptives, noncontraceptive estrogens, and other factors. JAMA 242:1150–1154
42. Report by the Management Committee (1980) The Australian Therapeutic Trial in Mild Hypertension. Lancet 1:1261–1267

43. Rubens J, Espeland MA, Ryu J, Harpold G, McKinney WM, Kahl FR, Toole JF, Crouse III JR (1998) Individual variation in susceptibility to extracranial carotid atherosclerosis. Arteriosclerosis 8:389–397
44. Schnall PL, Alderman MH, Kern R (1984) An analysis of the HDFP trial. Evidence of adverse effects of antihypertensive treatment on white women with moderate and severe hypertension. N Y State Med J 84:299–301
45. SHEP Cooperative Research Group (1991) Prevention of stroke by antihypertensive drug treatment in older persons with isolated systolic hypertension. Final results of the Systolic Hypertension in the Elderly Program (SHEP). JAMA 265:3255–3264
46. Staessen J, Bulpitt CJ, Fagard R, Lijnen P, Amery A (1989) The influence of menopause on blood pressure. J Hum Hypertension 3:427–433
47. Stampfer MJ, Coldlitz GA, Willett WC, Manson JAE, Rosner B, Speizer FE, Hennekens CH (1991) Postmenopausal estrogen therapy and cardiovascular disease. Ten-year follow-up from the Nurses' Health Study. N Engl J Med 325:756–762
48. Stokes III J, Kannel WB, Wolf PA, D'Agostino RB, Cupples LA (1989) Blood pressure as a risk factor for cardiovascular disease. The Framingham Study – 30 years of follow-up. Hypertension 13[Suppl I]:I13–I18
49. The Fifth Report of the Joint National Committee on Detection, Evaluation, and Treatment of High Blood Pressure (1993) U.S. Department of Health and Human Services. Public Health Service. National Institutes of Health. NIH Publ No 93–1088
50. The Management Committee of the Australian National Blood Pressure Study (1984) Prognostic factors in the treatment of mild hypertension. Circulation 69:668–674
51. Systolic Hypertension in the Elderly Program (SHEP) Cooperative Research Group (1988) Rationale and design of a randomized clinical trial on prevention of stroke in isolated systolic hypertension. J Clin Epidemiol 41:1197–1208
52. WHO Monica Project (1988) Geographical variation in the major risk factors of coronary heart disease in men and women aged 35–64 years. World Health Stat Q 41:115–140
53. Tyroler HA, Heyden S, Bartel A, Cassel J, Cornoni JC, Hames CG, Kleinbaum D (1971) Blood pressure and cholesterol as coronary heart disease risk factors. Arch Intern Med 128:907–914
54. Van Berensteyn ECH, Van 'T Hof MA, De Waard H (1989) Contributions of ovarian failure and aging to blood pressure in normotensive perimenopausal women: a mixed longitudinal study. Am J Epidemiol 129:947–955
55. Veterans Administration Cooperative Study Group on Antihypertensive Agents (1970) Effects of treatment on morbidity in hypertension. Results in patients with diastolic blood pressure averaging 90 through 114 mmHg. JAMA 213:1145–1182
56. Weiss NS (1972) Relationship of menopause to serum cholesterol and arterial pressure: the United States Health Examination Survey of Adults. Am J Epidemiol 96:237–241
57. Williams JK, Adams MR, Herrington DM, Clarkson TB (1992) Short-term administration of estrogen and vascular responses of atherosclerotic coronary arteries. J Am Coll Cardiol 20:452–457
58. Yusuf S, Thom T, Abbott RD (1989) Changes in hypertension treatment and in congestive heart failure mortality in the United States. Hypertension 13[Suppl I]:I74–I79

Printing: Mercedesdruck, Berlin
Binding: Buchbinderei Lüderitz & Bauer, Berlin